Manual of Urodynamics for Gynaecologists

T0134306

Previous edition published by RCOG Press under the title Urodynamics Illustrated, 2011

Manual of Urodynamics for Gynaecologists

Edited by

Ranee Thakar
Croydon University Hospital

Philip Toozs-Hobson
Birmingham Women's Hospital

Lucia Dolan
Belfast City Hospital

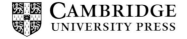
CAMBRIDGE
UNIVERSITY PRESS

CAMBRIDGE
UNIVERSITY PRESS

University Printing House, Cambridge CB2 8BS, United Kingdom

One Liberty Plaza, 20th Floor, New York, NY 10006, USA

477 Williamstown Road, Port Melbourne, VIC 3207, Australia

314–321, 3rd Floor, Plot 3, Splendor Forum, Jasola District Centre, New Delhi – 110025, India

79 Anson Road, #06–04/06, Singapore 079906

Cambridge University Press is part of the University of Cambridge.

It furthers the University's mission by disseminating knowledge in the pursuit of education, learning, and research at the highest international levels of excellence.

www.cambridge.org
Information on this title: www.cambridge.org/9781108432221
DOI: 10.1017/9781108346351

© Cambridge University Press 2020

First published 2020

Printed in Singapore by Markono Print Media Pte Ltd

A catalogue record for this publication is available from the British Library.

Library of Congress Cataloging-in-Publication Data
Names: Thakar, Ranee, editor. | Toozs-Hobson, Philip M., editor. | Dolan, Lucia, editor.
Title: Manual of urodynamics for gynaecologists / edited by Ranee Thakar, Philip Toozs-Hobson, Lucia Dolan.
Description: Cambridge, United Kingdom ; New York, NY : Cambridge University Press, 2020. | Includes bibliographical references and index.
Identifiers: LCCN 2019038912 (print) | LCCN 2019038913 (ebook) | ISBN 9781108432221 (paperback) | ISBN 9781108346351 (epub)
Subjects: MESH: Urodynamics–physiology | Patient Reported Outcome Measures
Classification: LCC RC900 (print) | LCC RC900 (ebook) | NLM WJ 102 | DDC 616.6–dc23
LC record available at https://lccn.loc.gov/2019038912
LC ebook record available at https://lccn.loc.gov/2019038913

ISBN 978-1-108-43222-1 Paperback

Additional resources for this publication at www.cambridge.org/ 9781108432221.

Contents

Contributors

Paul Abrams

Kate Anders

Nikki Cotterill

Prathiba De Silva

Marcus Drake

Chris Harding

Emmanuel Karantanis

Reeba Oliver

Ivilina Pandeva

Matthew Parsons

Kal Perkins

Smita Rajshekhar

Angie Rantell

Ahmed Shaban

Mark Slack

Sushma Srikrishna

Lucy Swithinbank

Ranee Thakar

Laura Thomas

Louise Webster

Preface

We are grateful for the continued support of many of the authors for their updated chapters and also grateful for the support of the old authors who have retired or left practice for their help in enlisting new authors.

Urodynamics has been under increased scrutiny in its utility. Since the 1st Edition the The National Institute For Health and Care Excellence (NICE) guidelines for healthcare professionals have been updated and a new version of the Minimum Standards for Urodynamics from United Kingdom Continence Society (UKCS) has been published. In response, we have included a chapter incorporating those revised standards for urodynamics. It is important that if a test is to be performed then it should be performed to the highest standards. We hope that you will have acquired the knowledge to enable you when you have finished reading this book.

Preface to Urodynamics Illustrated

This book provides concise information to help clinicians who are new to urodynamics as well as acting as an aide-memoire for established practitioners. It was born out of the recognised need for a manual that can be an instant reference for practitioners. The book follows many of the key principles taught on the joint Royal College of Obstetricians and Gynaecologists and British Society of Urogynaecology Urodynamics Course and uses the *Minimum Standards in Urodynamics* document and the International Continence Society standards as the main underpinning documentation for the text [1, 2].

We cannot overstate the importance of the expertise of the observer when attempting to obtain accurate and reliable measurements when performing urodynamics. Good urodynamic practice occurs when there is a clear urodynamic question, adequate patient preparation, appropriate technical expertise and an interactive test. In this book, we provide both a technical and clinical guide for the urodynamics observer through illustration of many of the practical steps and common clinical observations reported in the urodynamics laboratory. Several urodynamic investigations are discussed, ranging from the basic tests such as uroflowmetry and subtracted cystometry to the more complex, namely videocystometry, ambulatory monitoring and urethral function tests. The key principles of measurement of physiological and pathophysiological parameters of lower urinary tract function are common, irrespective of type of investigation. This book should provide the core knowledge to undertake these measurements and an understanding of their limitations. Much of the information described for setting up equipment acts as a general guide when getting started and troubleshooting during investigation.

It is essential that these invasive, embarrassing tests are undertaken by clinicians who interpret the results in the context of symptoms rather than in isolation. The main learning points are summarised at the end of each chapter and guidance on avoidance of urodynamic pitfalls is provided within the chapter on artefacts. A selection of clinical cases has been included in many chapters to place the investigations within the context of a symptom complex. These examples and the core text should provide the key knowledge for everyday practice. However, it behoves us to say that true expertise will come from experiential learning and regular urodynamic practice. For the first time, the role and responsibilities of those undertaking urodynamics and those in training have been defined [1].

Finally, we hope that you will keep this book in your urodynamics laboratory as an easy reference and, when you have outgrown its pages, that you will use it as an illustrative text for teaching others the fundamentals of good urodynamic practice.

References

1. Association for Continence Advice, British Association of Paediatric Urologists, British Association of Urological Nurses, British Association of Urological Surgeons, British Society of Urogynaecology, Chartered Society of Physiotherapists, Royal College of Nursing Continence Care Forum, United Kingdom Continence

Society, Urogynaecology Nurse Specialists Network. *Joint Statement on Minimum Standards for Urodynamic Practice in the UK. Prepared by a working party.* UK Continence Society; 2009 [www.ukcs.uk .net].

2. Schäfer W, Abrams P, Liao L, Mattiasson A, Pesce F, Spangberg A, et al. Good urodynamic practices: uroflowmetry, filling, cystometry, and pressure-flow studies. *Neurourol Urodyn.* 2002;21:261–74.

Pre-test Assessment of Urinary Dysfunction, Using Patient-Centred Questionnaires

Nikki Cotterill

1.1 The History of the Development of Patient-Centred Questionnaire Assessment

Patient-centred questionnaires and patient-reported outcome (PRO) measures are terms that are used interchangeably to reflect an instrument that provides evaluation of the lived experience of symptoms from the patients' perspective. PRO use has grown significantly in the past 10–15 years, due to recognition of the importance of placing patients at the centre of their care [1]. It is recognised that only those individuals *experiencing* symptoms can report on the more subjective elements [2]. This is particularly important in the case of urodynamics, which is a clinical test. PROs provide a method of measuring subjective phenomena in an objective way and provide context to the data provided by clinical measurements. PROs can be used to record the presence and severity of symptoms and also to measure their impact, in particular on quality of life. This is useful when interpreting patients' priorities for treatment and understanding the most bothersome aspect of their symptoms.

PROs must be developed using a robust methodology in order to provide accurate measurements. It is therefore necessary to understand the principles underpinning their development in order to select the most appropriate questionnaires to use for a given patient, condition or clinical intervention [3]. The key characteristics to determine the robustness of a PRO are as follows (summarised in Table 1.1):

- Context of use – the intended population.
- Content validity – the process of item generation and interpretation of the PRO.
- Psychometric robustness – characteristics of the measurement properties. (FDA 2009, www.fda.gov/regulatory-information/search-fda-guidance-documents/patient-reported-outcome-measures-use-medical-product-development-support-labeling-claims)

1.1.1 Context of Use

The PRO should be developed in a population that represents the intended respondents, to promote its applicability [4]. The developmental population may be specific and the appropriateness of the PRO for the intended population should be evaluated. Where the PRO appears to be relevant but has not been developed in the specific population, it can be further evaluated in the intended population for its relevance and appropriateness. The important factor is whether input has been sought from the intended population to derive the PRO content. Only by conducting qualitative research, for example, through interviews or focus groups, can the PRO be capture issues of relevance that are pertinent to potential respondents.

Table 1.1 PRO characteristics to evaluate measurement capability and robustness

Parameter	Importance in PRO selection
Context of use	Determines appropriateness for the population in which use is intended
Content validity	Evidence of comprehensiveness and relevance to the population, and interpretation by potential respondents
Psychometric robustness • *Additional validity* • *Reliability* • *Responsiveness*	Quantitative data that provide evidence of measurement capability to provide robust and accurate data

1.1.2 Content Validity

Content validity is an evaluation of whether the PRO captures what it intends to measure and whether it can be clearly interpreted to provide these data [2,5]. Cognitive debriefing interviews are typically employed to evaluate this in which potential respondents complete the draft PRO and discuss their thoughts while completing the tool, followed by a structured interview to assess whether question items are interpreted as intended [6].

1.1.3 Psychometric Robustness

1.1.3.1 Additional Validity

Other components of validity testing include:

- Convergent validity – quantitative assessment of the relationship between findings from the PRO and measures of similar variables. Where constructs are closely related, the relationships should be stronger, and weaker relationships evident with more poorly related constructs.
- Discriminant validity – an assessment of the PRO's capability to distinguish between known patient groups, for example, those with mild, moderate, and severe symptoms.
- Criterion validity – an assessment of the relationship between the PRO and an accepted gold standard, if available. Clinical proxy measures can be used as a direct comparison with a PRO, due to its variable nature is rarely possible.

These elements are typically considered essential for the complete validation of a PRO but should be judged in context. The more components of validity evaluated will provide more evidence of the robustness of the PRO to provide accurate and reliable data.

1.1.3.2 Reliability

The ability of the PRO to measure in a consistent manner over time is vital to ensure any change detected is due to a real change in symptom status, rather than measurement error. This can be measured in two ways:

- Internal consistency – a measure of the homogeneity of the questionnaire or how well the items relate to each other, without a direct duplication.
- Test–retest reliability – a measure of the stability of responses over time when symptom status is considered to have remained stable.

1.1.3.3 Responsiveness

The PRO's ability to detect change where real symptom improvement, or deterioration, has occurred is particularly important for outcome measurement in order to evaluate the change following intervention. The magnitude of change should also be evident in order to make comparisons between treatments with anticipated different effect sizes; for example, surgical versus conservative intervention [1].

1.2 The International Consultation on Incontinence Modular Questionnaire (ICIQ)

1.2.1 An ICIQ Overview

The International Consultation on Incontinence Modular Questionnaire (ICIQ) was developed to provide a universally applicable, standardised series of self-completion assessment instruments to evaluate lower urinary tract symptoms, lower bowel symptoms and vaginal symptoms [7]. It began in 1999 and now consists of a collection of 16 high-quality questionnaires including a validated bladder diary [8,9].

The ICIQ PROs can be used by men and women irrespective of age, with varied causes for their symptoms, facilitating the use of common questionnaires in many patient groups. It was developed from a standard protocol for the development and translation of ICIQ questionnaires. The content of the questionnaires is derived from patients and clinical experts, providing a robust evidence base for inclusion.

Core modules evaluate the core symptoms of lower pelvic dysfunction, namely lower urinary tract, lower bowel and vaginal symptoms. An example of an ICIQ module, the ICIQ-UI Short Form, is provided in Figure 1.1.

Additional specialised and detailed modules are available, such as overactive bladder symptoms, nocturia, quality of life and sexual matters (Table 1.2).

The ICIQ is an international collaborative project encouraging worldwide standardisation of assessment and is available in numerous languages. Collaboration is invited to further develop questionnaires and translations.

1.2.2 Use of the ICIQ

A number of ICIQ modules have now been incorporated into The National Institute of Health and Care Excellence (NICE) guidelines with recommendations for their use when evaluating interventions and recognition of their status in the field of PRO provision [10]. In Scotland, primary care guidelines include recommendations for use of the ICIQ [11]. They are recommended as first line for PROs and global use in clinical practice and research by the triennial international consultation on incontinence [1]. Questionnaire modules are supplied free of charge for clinical practice and academic research. They can be accessed via the project website www.iciq.net.

With the need to provide electronic patient records, the requirement to move away from paper and pencil administration is increasingly recognised. The eICIQ has been fully validated to provide evidence of the equivalence of its measurement properties in the altered format and its online provision is in development [12].

ICIQ-UI Short Form

CONFIDENTIAL

Initial number

DAY   MONTH   YEAR
Today's date

Many people leak urine some of the time. We are trying to find out how many people leak urine, and how much this bothers them. We would be grateful if you could answer the following questions, thinking about how you have been, on average, over the PAST FOUR WEEKS.

1 Please write in your date of birth:

DAY   MONTH   YEAR

2 Are you *(tick one)*:   Female ☐   Male ☐

3 How often do you leak urine? *(Tick one box)*

never ☐	0
about once a week or less often ☐	1
two or three times a week ☐	2
about once a day ☐	3
several times a day ☐	4
all the time ☐	5

4 We would like to know how much urine <u>you think</u> leaks.
How much urine do you <u>usually</u> leak (whether you wear protection or not)?
(Tick one box)

none ☐	0
a small amount ☐	2
a moderate amount ☐	4
a large amount ☐	6

5 Overall, how much does leaking urine interfere with your everyday life?
Please ring a number between 0 (not at all) and 10 (a great deal)

0   1   2   3   4   5   6   7   8   9   **10**
not at all   a great deal

ICIQ score: sum scores 3+4+5 ☐☐

6 When does urine leak? *(Please tick all that apply to you)*

never – urine does not leak	☐
leaks before you can get to the toilet	☐
leaks when you cough or sneeze	☐
leaks when you are asleep	☐
leaks when you are physically active/exercising	☐
leaks when you have finished urinating and are dressed	☐
leaks for no obvious reason	☐
leaks all the time	☐

Thank you very much for answering these questions.

Figure 1.1 ICIQ-UI Short Form (© ICIQ group). See www.iciq.net for ICIQ user policy: questionnaires can be requested centrally for supply in their original format

Table 1.2 The International Consultation on Incontinence Modular Questionnaire structure

Condition	Recommended modules	Optional modules	Recommended add-on modules		
	(A) Core modules		QoL	Sexual matters	Post-treatment
Urinary symptoms	Males: ICIQ-MLUTS Females: ICIQ-FLUTS	Males: ICIQ-MLUTS LF Females: ICIQ-FLUTS LF	ICIQ-LUTSqol	Males: ICIQ-MLUTSsex Females: ICIQ-FLUTSsex	ICIQ-S[a] (satisfaction)
	ICIQ-bladder diary				
Vaginal symptoms	ICIQ-VS		ICIQ-VSqol[a]		
Bowel symptoms	ICIQ-B	ICIQ-IBD			
Urinary incontinence	ICIQ-UI SF	ICIQ-UI LF[a]	ICIQ-LUTSqol	Males: ICIQ-MLUTSsex Females: ICIQ-FLUTSsex	
Condition	(B) Specific patient groups		QoL	Sexual matters	
Nocturia	ICIQ-N		ICIQ-Nqol	Males: ICIQ-MLUTSsex Females: ICIQ-FLUTSsex	
Overactive bladder	ICIQ-OAB		ICIQ-OABqol	Males: ICIQ-MLUTSsex Females: ICIQ-FLUTSsex	
Underactive bladder	ICIQ-UAB[a]				
Long-term catheter	ICIQ-LTCqol				
Children	ICIQ-CLUTS[a]				
Absorbent pads			ICIQ-Padprom		
Cognitively impaired adults	ICIQ-Cognitively impaired adults[a]				

[a] Developmental version in process of validation.

1.3 Other Recommended Questionnaires for LUTS and Quality of Life Assessment

Whilst the ICIQ is the PRO of choice, it is recognised that these questionnaires may not be appropriate for an intended purpose [13]. Grade A recommendations are awarded where there is published evidence of validity, reliability and responsiveness according to standard psychometric testing. If additional evidence of content validity evaluation is provided, a Grade A* is awarded to reflect the extra efforts taken to ensure the most rigorous developmental processes were undertaken at the item generation stage.

1.4 Advantages and Disadvantages of Using Patient-Centred Questionnaires

PROs offer valuable patient insight into the lived experience of their symptoms and their use is advocated in clinical practice and research globally. It is important to be aware of their strengths and limitations, particularly for their inclusion in clinical practice, as identified below.

Advantages
- Quick and comprehensive assessment of symptoms and associated 'bother'.
- Complement clinical assessment of patients with lower urinary tract symptoms.
- Valuable for evaluating outcomes of treatment or interventions.
- Provides a vehicle to raise the discussion about symptoms often considered embarrassing and which patients are often reluctant to disclose.
- Provides the patients' perspective of their symptoms and a measure of their severity.
- Relatively cheap method of data collection although must consider associated costs such as administration and data entry.
- Provides a robust tool for clinical audit and research.

Disadvantages
- PROs must be used as intended and proxy completion can be inaccurate if this method of completion has not been evaluated.
- PROS can be restrictive in their remit and format and prevent patients from providing further information.
- Patients may inadvertently skew data to provide 'false positive' perspectives to conform with socially accepted norms, or 'false negative' perspectives that exaggerate the severity of their symptoms.
- Postal response rates can be poor.
- Translation availability may restrict the populations able to complete PROs.
- Data may be missing due to PRO questions being overlooked.
- Due to the subjective nature of the assessment, the current status of the patient may alter the answers provided.

1.5 Access to Patient-Centred Questionnaires

Aside from contacting individual authors, there are a number of ways to access PROs through collection databases. Larger projects such as the ICIQ can be accessed directly through the project website, given the nature of the project and number of questionnaires available. Industry developers also host database collections of their tools such as the Pfizer

Patient-Reported Outcomes platform: www.pfizerpatientreportedoutcomes.com. ProQolid is an independent database of clinical outcome assessments that is organised by symptom area to provide an overview of measures available and their characteristics in order to make informed choices and provide access routes to individual PROs (https://eprovide.mapi-trust.org/about/about-proqolid). Licences and fees may apply according to the intended use, which should be established before implementation in the clinical or research setting. *ePAQ (electronic Personal Assessment Questionnaire)* is a validated, web-based clinical assessment system, specifically designed to provide detailed self-reported symptoms and quality of life data from women with pelvic floor disorders. ePAQ enables the delivery of virtual clinics and provides valuable outcomes data for activities including audit, service evaluation, revalidation, appraisal and research [14].

References

1. Castro-Diaz D, Robinson D, Bosch R, et al. Patient-reported outcome assessment. *Incontinence: Proceedings of the Sixth International Consultation on Incontinence*, Tokyo, September 2016. Plymouth: Health Publications Limited; 2017: 541–670.

2. Streiner DL, Norman GR, Cairney J. *Health Measurement Scales: A Practical Guide to Their Development and Use.* Oxford University Press; 2014:415.

3. Donovan J, Bosch R, Gotoh M, et al. Symptom and quality of life assessment. *Incontinence: Proceedings of the Third International Consultation on Incontinence*, Paris, June 2004. Plymouth: Health Publications Limited; 2005:519–84.

4. Food and Drug Administration (FDA). *Guidance for Industry Patient-Reported Outcome Measures: Use in Medical Product Development to Support Labeling Claims*; 2014.

5. Oppenheim A. *Questionnaire Design, Interviewing and Attitude Measurement.* 2nd edition. London: Continnuum-3PL; 1998:312.

6. Patrick DL, Burke LB, Gwaltney CJ, et al. Content validity – establishing and reporting the evidence in newly developed patient-reported outcomes (PRO) instruments for medical product evaluation: ISPOR PRO good research practices task force report: part 1 – eliciting concepts for a new PRO instrument. *Value Health J Int Soc Pharmacoeconomics Outcomes Res.* 2011;14:967–77.

7. Abrams P, Avery K, Gardener N, Donovan J, ICIQ Advisory Board. The International Consultation on Incontinence Modular Questionnaire: www.iciq.net. *J Urol.* 2006;175:1063–6; discussion 1066.

8. Bright E, Cotterill N, Drake M, Abrams P. Developing a validated urinary diary: phase 1. *Neurourol Urodyn.* 2012;31:625–33.

9. Bright E, Cotterill N, Drake M, Abrams P. Developing and validating the International Consultation on Incontinence Questionnaire bladder diary. *Eur Urol.* 2014;66(2):294–300.

10. National Institute for Health and Care Excellence. Urinary incontinence in women: management. NICE Guideline (CG171); 2013.

11. Scottish Intercollegiate Guidelines Network. Management of urinary incontinence in primary care; 2004.

12. Uren AD, Cotterill N, Parke SE, Abrams P. Psychometric equivalence of electronic and telephone completion of the ICIQ modules. *Neurourol Urodyn.* 2016;36:1342–1349.

13. Abrams P, Cardozo L, Wagg A, Wein A. *Incontinence: Proceedings of the Sixth International Consultation on Incontinence*, Tokyo, 2016. Plymouth: Health Publications Limited; 2017.

14. Jones GL, Radley SC, Lumb J, Farkas A. Responsiveness of the electronic Personal Assessment Questionnaire-Pelvic Floor (ePAQ-PF). *Int Urogynecol J Pelvic Floor Dysfunct.* 2009;20:557–64.

The Assessment of Women with Lower Urinary Tract Dysfunction, Using Bladder Diaries

Prathiba De Silva and Matthew Parsons

A bladder diary provides an objective evaluation of the severity of urinary storage symptoms and associated urinary incontinence. Bladder diaries are not used to diagnose detrusor overactivity or urodynamic stress incontinence; however, they help to guide conservative management and to provide lifestyle advice, and keeping a bladder diary is the only method available to diagnose nocturnal polyuria.

2.1 Types

- *Frequency-volume chart* (FVC) – records the volumes voided and the times of each micturition during day and night, over at least 24 hours.
- *Bladder diary* (BD) or *voiding diary* – records micturition times, voided volumes, incontinence episodes, pad usage and other information such as fluid intake, the degree of urgency and the degree of incontinence [1].

2.2 Features

- Bladder diaries should be completed as a mandatory part of the basic assessment of urinary incontinence, prior to treatment as recommended by NICE [2].
- They are more accurate than recall when recording urinary symptoms and are cheap and easy to use.
- They can guide many aspects of conservative treatment, and inform timing and type of fluid intake.
- Non-completion of a diary does not exclude urinary symptoms.
- Reduction in bladder capacity and 24-hour voided volume is associated with aging.
- Ideally, a bladder diary should include a minimum of 3 days, covering variations in usual activities, such as both working and leisure days [3,4].
- They are especially useful in identifying the following:
  - disorders associated with compulsive/excessive fluid intake, e.g., diabetes insipidus/mellitus, habitual excessive intake;
  - inappropriate normal fluid consumption (e.g., at bedtime causing nocturia);
  - excessive intake of alcohol or caffeine causing exacerbation of symptoms.
- Learned or habitual frequency may only be semi-objectively assessed.

2.3 Information Provided by a Bladder Diary

- Functional bladder capacity.
- 24-hour diurnal and nocturnal frequency of micturitions.

Birmingham Women's **NHS**
NHS Foundation Trust

Figure 2.1 **Paper diary**

Frequency Volume Chart

Time	Day 1 In	Day 1 Out	Day 1 Wet	Day 2 In	Day 2 Out	Day 2 Wet	Day 3 In	Day 3 Out	Day 3 Wet
7 am		340					260		
8 am	300			400	330		350		
9 am		200						170	
10 am	200	150		150	200		200		
11 am			W		175			150	
12 pm		200		150				50	
1 pm	150			150	200	W	320	200	
2 pm		175					320	200	
3 pm				200				200	
4 pm	450	150			220				W
5 pm		100					150		
6 pm		100	W	300			150	175	
7 pm	250	175		500	200 150				
8 pm	200	50		400	150 150	W	450	100	
9 pm	100				50	W		100	W
10 pm	350	180	860	150			400	200	
11 pm					210	860		210	860
12 am									
1 am		270					200		
2 am	100					W			
3 am		300							
4 am					210				
5 am									
6 am									

- Daytime micturitions defined as voiding during waking hours and includes the last void before sleep and the first void after waking.
- Nocturia is the number of voids recorded during a night sleep: each void is preceded and followed by sleep.
- Voided volumes during the daytime and during the night (which assumes voiding immediately after rising in the morning, and before going to bed).
- Duration of day and night, to allow calculation of production rates including nocturnal polyuria which includes the morning void in the nighttime production.

2.4 Formats for Diaries

2.4.1 Paper

This is the most common format (see Figure 2.1).

Advantages

- Easily posted or handed directly to the patient.
- Easy to produce.
- Inexpensive to post.
- Easily and safely stored.

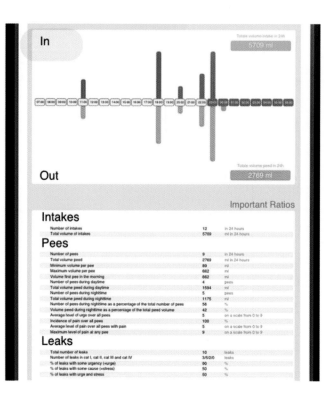

Figure 2.2 iP voidingdiary™

Disadvantages

- 24-hour and nocturnal total volumes are manually calculated which is time-consuming and inaccuracies may occur.
- Strong positive relationship between bladder capacity and 24-hour voided volume is not accounted for (unlike an electronic diary).
- Strong negative relationship with age, in normality and detrusor overactivity, is not accounted for [5,6].
- 'Eye-balling' charts may therefore lead to inaccuracy.

2.4.2 Electronic

Advantages

- Digital format can be recorded onto a computer, tablet or even smart phone.
- Patients find more user-friendly as it is quicker and more convenient than carrying a paper diary [7].
- It allows for centile rankings correcting for age and 24-hour voided volume, generating a customised report that is not provided by paper formats (see Figure 2.2) [8].

Disadvantages

- Lack of visualisation of the voiding pattern on 3-day diary.
- Inability to change mistakes made by the patient during completion [9].

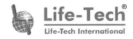

BLADDER DIARY RESULTS

Patient:		**Calculation Parameters**	
Patient ID	BW000	Volumes prorated:	Yes
Age:	51 **years**	Percentile calculation:	Adjust for age and volume
Sex:	F	**Diary Duration (Hours)**	69.6
Physician:		**Start Date**	12/12/2008

Frequency-Volume Data

Per 24 Hours	Amount	Percentile
Frequency (voids)	8.0	57%
Total Volume (ml)	2367	80%
Production Rate (ml/min)	1.64	79%

Volume Per Void (ml)	Amount	Percentile
Minimum	100	68%
Maximum	600	47%
Average	273	37%
Range	500	24%

	Day		Night	
Day vs Night	**Amount**	**Percentile**	**Amount**	**Percentile**
Frequency (voids)	7.9	55%	0.3	60%
Total Volume (ml)	2025	89%	342	29%
Production Rate (ml/min)	2.01	85%	0.79	31%
Production Rate % of 24H	123%	80%	48%	11%

Incontinence Episodes

Average Number of Episodes per 24 Hours	3.9	**Percent Caused by Activity**	40%
Average Leak Size Score (Scale1–3)	1.5	**Percent Accompanied by Urge**	70%

Frequency-Volume Chart

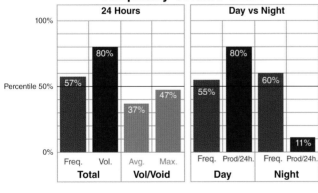

Figure 2.3 Bladder diary of a woman with USI

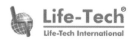

BLADDER DIARY RESULTS

Patient:

		Calculation Parameters	
Patient ID	1003	Volumes prorated:	Yes
Age:	59 years	Percentile calculation:	Adjust for age and volume
Sex:	F	**Diary Duration (Hours)**	47.7
Physician:		**Start Date**	11/01/2009

Frequency-Volume Data

Per 24 Hours	Amount	Percentile
Frequency (voids)	11.0	95%
Total Volume (ml)	2096	68%
Production Rate (ml/min)	1.46	69%

Volume Per Void (ml)	Amount	Percentile
Minimum	15	2%
Maximum	400	9%
Average	204	11%
Range	385	6%

	Day		Night	
Day vs Night	Amount	Percentile	Amount	Percentile
Frequency (voids)	8.6	84%	2.0	97%
Total Volume (ml)	1340	55%	756	88%
Production Rate (ml/min)	1.61	71%	1.25	70%
Production Rate % of 24H	110%	55%	86%	53%

Incontinence Episodes

Average Number of Episodes per 24 Hours	2.7	**Percent Caused by Activity**	0%
Average Leak Size Score (Scale1–3)	1.2	**Percent Accompanied by Urge**	20%

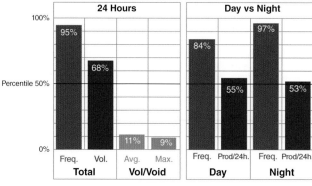

Figure 2.4 Bladder diary of a woman with DO

2.5 Bladder Diary Patterns

Detrusor overactivity (DO) patients tend to have the following when compared to urodynamic stress incontinence (USI) patients (see Figures 2.3 and 2.4) [10,11]:

1. higher voiding frequency;
2. lower volume/void;
3. more urge-related, than activity-related, leaks;
4. smaller volume, and equally frequent leaks;
5. more severe incontinence symptoms.

References

1. Bo K, Frawley HC, Haylen BT, et al. An International Urogynecological Association (IUGA)/International Continence Society (ICS) joint report on the terminology for the conservative and nonpharmacological management of female pelvic floor dysfunction. *Neurourol Urodyn.* 2017;36:221–4.

2. National Institute for Health and Care Excellence (NICE). Urinary incontinence: the management of urinary incontinence in women. NICE Guideline [CG171]; 2013. Available from www.nice.org.uk/guidance/cg171/evidence/urinary-incontinence-in-women-full-guideline-191581165. Accessed 26 March 2018.

3. Groutz A, Blaivas JG, Chaikin DC, et al. Noninvasive outcome measures of urinary incontinence and lower urinary tract symptoms: a multicenter study of micturition diary and pad tests. *J Urol.* 2000;164:698–701.

4. Syan R, Brucker BM. Guidelines of guidelines: urinary incontinence. *BJU Int.* 2015;117(1):20–3.

5. Amundsen CL, Parsons M, Tissot B, Cardozo L, Diokno A, Coats AC. Bladder diary measurements in asymptomatic females: functional bladder capacity, frequency and 24-hr volume. *Neurourol Urodyn.* 2007;26:341–9.

6. Parsons M, Tissot W, Cardozo L, Diokno A, Amundsen CL, Coats AC. Normative bladder diary measurements: night versus day. *Neurourol Urodyn.* 2007;26:465–73.

7. Abrams P, Paty J, Newgreen DT, et al. Electronic bladder diaries of differing duration versus a paper diary for data collection in overactive bladder. *Neurourol Urodyn.* 2016;35:743–9.

8. iP Voiding Diary. Available from www.synappz.nl/portfolio-item/ip-voiding-diary/?lang=en. Accessed 26 March 2018.

9. Mangera A, Marzo A, Heron N, et al. Development of two electronic bladder diaries: a patient and healthcare professionals pilot study. *Neurourol Urodyn.* 2014;33:1101–9.

10. Parsons M, Amundsen CL, Vella M, Webster GD, Coats AC. Bladder diary patterns in detrusor overactivity and urodynamic stress incontinence. *Neurourol Urodyn.* 2007;26:800–6.

11. Amundsen CL, Parsons M, Cardozo L, Vella M, Webster GD, Coats AC. Bladder diary volume per void measurements in detrusor overactivity. *J Urol.* 2006;176:2530–4.

Chapter 3

Pad Testing in the Assessment of Urinary Incontinence in Women

Emmanuel Karantanis

3.1 Introduction

Pad testing, most often used as an objective assessment of urinary incontinence, involves the use of pre-weighed continence pads to capture urinary leakage over a period of time. On completion of the tests, the pads are then weighed to calculate the amount of leakage.

3.2 Why Are Pad Tests Performed?

Pad tests are most commonly used in the research setting but can be an important clinical aid, especially in cases where it is uncertain that the 'leakage' is urinary in origin. Generally, pad tests are employed:

- To provide objective confirmation of urinary incontinence before and after treatment.
- To measure objectively the quantity of urine loss as a measure of severity: a 24-hour pad test loss of greater than 75 g represents severe incontinence in women with stress urinary incontinence [1].
- As a general aid when determining the type of incontinence: women with pure stress urinary incontinence have been shown to leak less than 100 g in 24 hours and those with overactive bladder have more severe leakage [1]; however, there is significant overlap, such that pad tests cannot be used to make an accurate diagnosis.
- To help to differentiate between urine and vaginal discharge in women who may have excessive vaginal fluid loss: urinary incontinence is unlikely if less than 2 g of loss is found on 24-hour pad test [2]; such tests should not be conducted with panty liners, as they have a tendency to evaporate their fluid.

3.3 Types of Pad Test

Pad testing methods differ with regard to duration (ranging between 1 and 72 hours) and in the activities undertaken during the test. The two most common methods used for pad testing are 1-hour and 24-hour tests.

3.3.1 One-Hour Pad Testing

One-hour pad tests are performed in a clinical setting, under the supervision of a continence nurse or doctor. They include a filling phase, during which the patient spends 15 minutes drinking 500 ml of fluid. This is followed by a series of provocative manoeuvres, such as coughing and jumping, to try to stimulate urinary leakage. Pads are weighed before and at the end of the test. Pad loss greater than 1 g is designated as significant or a 'positive pad test' [3].

3.3.2 Twenty-Four-Hour Pad Testing

Twenty-four-hour tests are performed at home. Women are provided with a set of pads and advised not to modify their normal drinking or activities. The aim of such tests is to document leakage in a normal home environment. Pad loss greater than 4 g is designated as significant or a 'positive pad test'. The values for 24-hour pad test are classified as follows: mild (4–20 g/24 hour), moderate (21–74 g/24 hour), and severe (>75 g/24 hour) incontinence [3].

3.4 Performing a Pad Test

3.4.1 Equipment

There are three components needed to perform a pad test:

- pads;
- snap-lock bags (one per test) to keep moisture in (all pad wrapping and adhesives should be placed in the bag to maintain an accurate post-test recording);
- weighing scales: scales accurate to 0.1 g should be used.

3.4.2 One-Hour Pad Test

The ICS Standardisation Committee has set out a standard protocol for the 1-hour pad test [3].

1. Test is started without the patient voiding.
2. Pre-weighed pad or collecting device is put in place by the subject and the first 1-hour test period begins.
3. Subject is given 500 ml sodium-free liquid to drink within a short period (maximum 15 minutes) and then the subject sits or rests for 15 minutes.
4. Half-hour period: subject walks, including stair climbing equivalent to one flight up and down.
5. During the remaining period, the subject performs the following activities:

   i. standing up from sitting, 10 times;
   ii. coughing vigorously, 10 times;
   iii. running on the spot, 1 min;
   iv. bending to pick up a small object from floor, 5 times;
   v. wash hands in running water, 1 min.

6. At the end of the 1-hour test, the pad or collecting device is removed and weighed.
7. If the test is regarded as representative, the subject is asked to void and the voided volume is recorded.
8. If the test is not regarded as representative, the test is repeated, preferably without voiding.

3.4.3 Twenty-Four-Hour Pad Test

The 24-hour pad test has not been standardised. The following is a description of the 24-hour pad test as used by the author:

1. Women are provided with five incontinence pads (such as Tena Lady Normal™, SCA Hygiene Products, Göteborg, Sweden; these pads are less evaporative than panty liners, less absorptive than thicker pads and more accurately reflect the fluid deposited on them).
2. Each pad is pre-weighed within a snap-lock bag. Women start the test in the morning and change to a new pad every 4 hours during the day. Whenever a pad is removed, it must be reinserted in its original snap-lock bag together with the wrappings and adhesives that were originally weighed. At the end of the day, the women wear their final pad for about 8 hours overnight and complete the test upon waking.
3. The pads are returned within 7 days, as they are shown to hold moisture if sealed [4].
4. Women do not need to undertake any particular provocative activities apart from their usual activities. It is useful to perform any vigorous activities that usually produce leakage activities while undertaking the test.
5. Twenty-four-hour pad tests are particularly informative when performed simultaneously with a bladder chart.

3.5 Comparison of 1-Hour and 24-Hour Pad Tests

The 24-hour pad test has been found to be repeatable and more sensitive than the 1-hour pad test in detecting urinary incontinence [5]. It requires fewer staff resources and less time and has been correlated with subjective severity measures [1,6–8]. The upper limit of normal for a 24-hour pad test is 2 g when using Tena Lady Normal™ pads. The report of the fourth International Consultation on Incontinence 2016 suggested that the 24-hour pad test was preferable because of the poor predictive value of the 1-hour pad test in the diagnosis of female urinary incontinence [5].

Clinical Scenario 1

A woman has constant moistness in the vagina, causing her to wear a pantyliner. The pantyliner tends to be damp but does not contain obvious significant amounts of urine. Despite this, the patient insists the panyliner smells like urine. In this case, the cause of the dampness could be urine or vaginal mucus. A 24-hour pad showing >4 g of loss would point towards a urinary loss.

Tip. Encouraging the woman to take Vitamin B complex tablets during the 24-hour pad test can be helpful because urine on the pantyliner ought to stain orange, and help confirm or negate whether urine is the cause of the dampness.

Clinical Scenario 2

A woman who leaks only during sport has a normal urodynamic assessment. Pelvic floor muscle training and the use of continence devices fail to control the leakage. The woman wants to proceed with surgery, but there is no objective evidence of urinary incontinence.

In this case, a 24-hour pad test conducted during a weekend of sport together with a bladder diary showing activity can confirm significant leakage during sport. Activity has been shown to increase 24-hour pad weight gain in women complaining of stress urinary incontinence [9].

3.6 Limitations of Pad Tests

- Not standardised.
- Results influenced by fluid intake, increased voiding difficulty, sweating, vaginal discharge.
- Inability to measure compliance.
- No diagnostic accuracy.
- No correlation to severity.

3.7 Summary

Pad tests are of most value in the research setting before and after treatment, as an objective endpoint of urinary incontinence. The activity undertaken by the women during a test may influence the results such that a similar level of activity should be performed when pad testing for comparison before and after treatment. Women's compliance with 24-hour pad tests decreases once cured. The same types of pad should be used for all patients before and after treatment, as pads have different absorptive and evaporative qualities. The major limitation of the pad test is the lack of diagnostic ability.

Learning Points

- Pad tests are most commonly used in the research and clinical settings as an objective endpoint of urinary incontinence.
- Pad test methodology varies in duration and type of activities undertaken, with 1-hour and 24-hour tests being the most common types.
- The same type of pad should be used throughout and Tena Lady Normal™ pads are the most suitable absorptive type.
- A positive 1-hour pad test is urine loss greater than 1 g and a positive 24-hour test is urine loss greater than 4 g.

References

1. O'Sullivan R, Karantanis E, Stevermuer TL, Allen W, Moore KH. Definition of mild, moderate and severe incontinence on the 24-hour pad test. *BJOG*. 2004;111:859–62.

2. Karantanis E, O'Sullivan R, Moore KH. The 24-hour pad test in continent women and men: normal values and cyclical alterations. *BJOG*. 2003;110:567–71.

3. Krhut J, Zachoval R, Smith PP, et al. Pad weight testing in the evaluation of urinary incontinence. *Neurourol Urodyn*. 2014;33:507–10.

4. Versi E, Orrego G, Hardy E, Seddon G, Smith P, Anand D. Evaluation of the home pad test in the investigation of female urinary incontinence. *BJOG*. 1996;103:162–7.

5. Abrams P, Cardozo L, Wagg A, Wein A (Eds). *Incontinence 6th Edition*. ICI-ICS. Bristol, UK: International Continence Society; 2017.

6. Costantini E, Lazzeri M, Bini V, Giannantoni A, Mearini L, Porena M. Sensitivity and specificity after one-hour pad test as a predictive value for female urinary incontinence. *Urol Int*. 2008;81:153–9.

7. Karantanis E, Allen W, Stevermeuer TL, Simons AM, O'Sullivan R, Moore KH. The repeatability of the 24-hour pad test. *Int Urogynecol J Pelvic Floor Dysfunct*. 2006;16:63–8.

8. Lose G, Jorgensen L, Thunedborg P. 24-hour home pad weighing test versus one-hour ward test in the assessment of mild stress incontinence. *Acta Obstet Gynecol Scand.* 1989;68:211–15.

9. Painter V, Karantanis E, Moore KH. Does patient activity level affect 24-hr pad test results in stress-incontinent women? *Neurourol Urodyn.* 2012;31:143–7.

Setting Up the Urodynamic Equipment

Lucy Swithinbank and Louise Webster

4.1 Introduction

Urodynamic equipment varies in complexity and a range of urodynamics machines are available. The choice of system depends on operator requirements. The *Buyers' Guide: Urodynamic Systems* by Centre for Evidence-Based Purchasing may help to inform choice [1,2].

4.2 The Urodynamics Laboratory

Guidelines have been published [3–5] and manufacturers normally provide training on any equipment purchased. The exact method of preparing equipment for a test varies. Calibration is generally best left to the service engineer or medical physics personnel and is usually undertaken as part of a service agreement.

4.3 Uroflowmetry Equipment

4.3.1 Flowmeter

There are two types of flowmeter that are commonly used: the rotating disc and the weight transducer. The rotating disc can be dismantled for cleaning. A stand-alone flowmeter may be used separately from cystometry.

4.3.2 Commode

A commode with a funnel is placed above the flowmeter to enable accurate aim of the flow on to the flowmeter (Figure 4.1).

4.4 Subtracted Cystometry Equipment

There are three methods, depending on whether pressure is measured using water-filled, solid-state or air-filled catheters. The equipment used for each method is described below.

4.4.1 Water-Filled System

The water-filled system is the current International Continence Society standard and is the most common method for cystometry [5]. External pressure transducers are mounted on the urodynamic equipment (Figure 4.2) and connected to the water-filled lines. The use of external transducers means that the system is prone to movement artefacts. The height of the transducers is adjusted when the patient's position changes relative to them. Water-

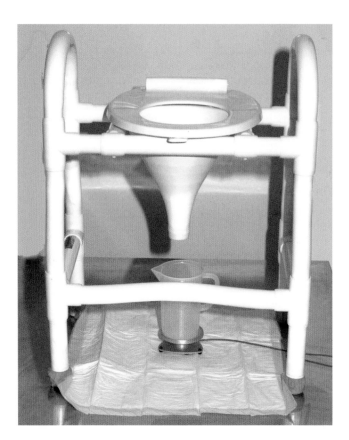

Figure 4.1 A flowmeter and commode

filled lines are prone to air bubbles collecting during the test. Lines should be flushed to expel air when there is damping, which would cause inaccurate measurement of pressure. The position of the syringes (superior, inferior or lateral) to the domes is unimportant as long as the principles of flushing through are followed.

4.4.1.1 Types of Water-Filled Catheters

A water-filled pressure catheter is placed in the bladder to measure intravesical pressure and a second catheter is inserted into either the rectum or the vagina to measure intra-abdominal pressure. Either single-lumen or double-lumen water-filled catheters can be used to measure intravesical pressure.

Single-Lumen Catheters

If a single-lumen catheter is chosen, a second catheter called the 'filling catheter' is inserted transurethrally alongside the vesical pressure catheter. The filling catheter is used to fill the bladder with saline and should be 8 Fr or less in diameter. The pressure catheter should be 4.5 Fr or less in diameter.

Double-Lumen Catheters

Double-lumen catheters have two lumens, with one lumen for filling with saline and one for measuring intravesical pressure. These are 6 or 8 Fr size and allow several filling and

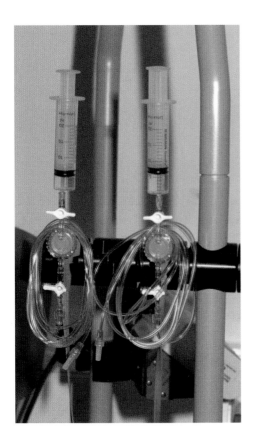

Figure 4.2 External pressure transducers mounted on the equipment

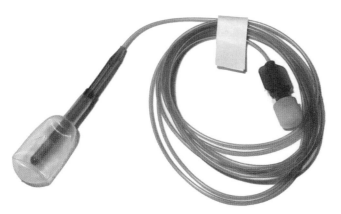

Figure 4.3 An abdominal catheter

voiding cycles. Double-lumen catheters with smaller gauge are more prone to pump artefacts when faster filling speeds are used.

Abdominal (Rectal/Vaginal) Catheters

Several prototypes of abdominal lines (Figure 4.3) are available from manufacturers.

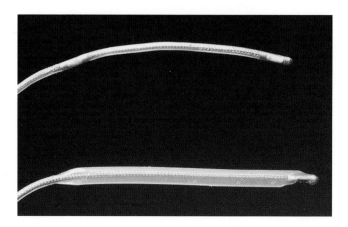

Figure 4.4 Solid-tip vesical catheter

4.4.2 Solid-State System

A solid-state catheter-tip transducer is not connected to an external pressure transducer because it has a transducer mounted at the tip of the catheter. This type of system is rarely used.

A filling catheter, similar to that used with a water-filled system, is inserted alongside the solid-tip catheter and is necessary to infuse water. Solid-tip vesical catheters (Figure 4.4) can be either a single transducer or a double transducer, which can be mounted to measure urethral pressure simultaneously.

Solid-state catheters with a single-tip transducer inserted into the rectum and covered with a condom, sheath or gloved finger can be used to measure intra-abdominal pressure.

4.4.3 Air-Filled Catheters

Air-filled catheters are disposable and have a valve that allows zeroing after catheterisation, but before priming of the balloon. Although they are commercially available, their use has not yet been validated. Recent studies have shown that pressures measured with air-filled catheters are not interchangeable with those using water-filled systems. Care should be taken when comparing results [6].

4.5 Other Equipment

Manometer tubing can be supplied by the manufacturer. It is used to connect catheters to transducers. Transducer pressure domes vary depending on the machine. In a water-filled system, domes are required to transfer water pressure to the transducers and protect the transducers when the equipment is not in use. Three-way taps are placed both above and below the domes to allow for zeroing and flushing the lines during the test [7]. The Medicines and Healthcare products Regulatory Agency (MHRA) has recommended that domes, manometer tubing and syringes be changed with each patient to prevent cross-infection [8]. This is costly and time-consuming and so some Trusts have introduced local rules concerning reuse.

Use latex-free disposables if a latex allergy is suspected.

4.6 Setting Up Uroflowmetry

The weight transducer flowmeter is placed on the floor under the commode and switched on. The rotating disc flowmeter is assembled by placing the disc above the motor and is then switched on. The funnel is placed in the commode and the commode is placed over the flowmeter.

Enter the patient's details on the urodynamics machine and then choose the uroflowmetry program from the menu on the machine. Recording starts when a flow is sensed automatically or when a 'start' button is pressed. The user should check the settings on the machine.

4.7 Setting Up Subtracted Dual-Channel Cystometry

Setting up can be considered as connecting the transducers and filling line and setting zero pressure. The technique for setting up will vary according to the type of system being used.

4.7.1 Connecting the Transducers

4.7.1.1 Water-Filled System

Dome covers are 'primed' by flushing with sterile water. This can be achieved by either pushing water through using prefilled syringes distally or 'pulling' water through the dome from a distal giving set and bag using an empty syringe proximal to the dome.

A tap should be placed between the syringe and the dome, as placing the tap in the 'off' position to the dome during measurement prevents damping of pressures, which might otherwise occur [7]. The different positions in which the taps are placed are important for flushing, zeroing and recording (Figure 4.5a).

4.7.1.2 Solid-State System

Since the transducers are sited on the catheter tip, the catheter cables are connected directly to the urodynamics equipment rather than to pressure domes.

4.7.1.3 Air-Filled Catheters

The interface cables should be connected to the urodynamics equipment. They should be left in the 'open' setting ready to connect with the catheters once inserted.

4.7.2 Connecting the Filling Line

The filling line is connected to a bag of infusion fluid, usually 0.9% physiological saline, suspended from a weighted transducer using pump-specific tubing, depending on the equipment.

4.7.3 Setting Zero Pressure

The transducers are set to atmospheric pressure, not to bladder or abdominal pressure. The method for zeroing is dependent on the choice of catheter (Figure 4.6).

4.7.3.1 Water-Filled System

When the selected programme on the urodynamic equipment has been chosen, the taps are turned so that they open to atmosphere. Press or select zero on the equipment.

(a)

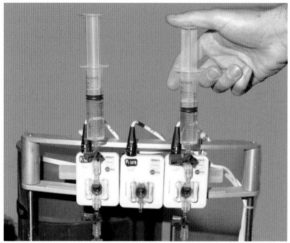

(b)

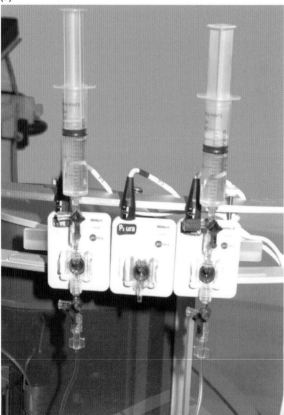

Figure 4.5 Three-way taps set for (a) flushing, (b) zeroing and (c) recording

(c)

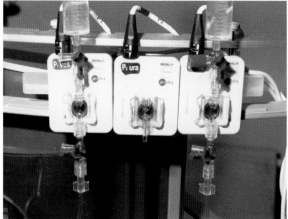

Figure 4.5 *(cont.)*

The 'zero' of the machine can be checked at any time during the test, if artefacts are suspected by turning the tap so that it is open to atmosphere. Connect the catheters to the equipment.

After catheterisation, the catheters should be flushed through the dome once they have been connected to remove any air bubbles. The external transducers are placed at the height of the superior aspect of the symphysis pubis as the reference level during recording.

4.7.3.2 Solid-State System

The catheters are connected to the equipment after sterilisation and then set to 'zero' while outside the patient and whilst maintaining sterility.

4.7.4 Air-Filled Catheters

The only air-filled catheter available at the time of publication uses a valve that can set the zero to atmospheric pressure even after catheterisation.

The equipment is now set to record the urodynamic test. Refer to Chapter 6 for information on performing the test, including how to maintain quality and troubleshoot during the investigation.

4.8 Maintenance of Calibration of Equipment

4.8.1 Checking Calibration

Calibration should be checked by users regularly. The timing of this procedure varies: every month is a good guide, unless there is concern about the accuracy of recorded measurements.

4.8.2 Checking Calibration of the Flowmeter

The flowmeter is calibrated using a constant-flow bottle. Water is poured into the flowmeter and the rate recorded and checked against the known constant flow rate. Alternatively, a

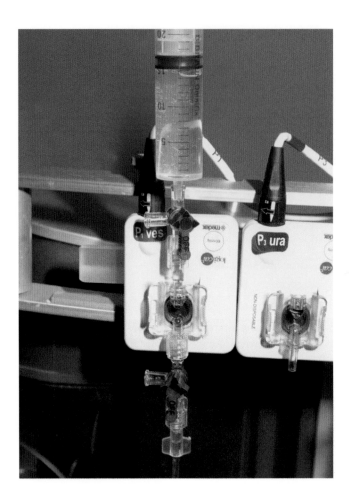

Figure 4.6 Zeroing the transducers to atmosphere with the taps open to atmosphere

recorded volume is checked by measuring the amount in the measuring jug against the volume recorded. This check is normally used instead of a constant-flow bottle.

4.8.3 Checking Calibration of the Urodynamic Machine

4.8.3.1 Water-Filled System

Zero the transducers with the taps open to atmosphere, and then, with the taps set for recording a test, place the tubing ends at the level of the external transducers. The pressure should read zero (Figure 4.7). The ends of the tubing are raised to a height of 50 or 100 cm measured against a ruler or marker. If the machine is correctly calibrated, the pressures should also read 50 or 100 cm H_2O on the equipment (Figure 4.8).

4.8.3.2 Solid-State Catheter-Tip Transducers

The calibration of solid-state catheter-tip transducers should also be checked regularly. This requires that the transducers are immersed to a set depth in water, rather than raised in air, or by means of a special calibration chamber which is capable of generating pressures in centimetres of water.

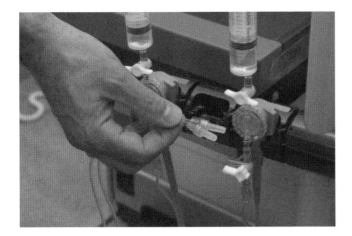

Figure 4.7 Checking zero with the tubing ends at the level of the external transducers

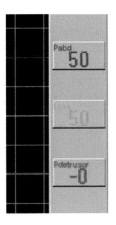

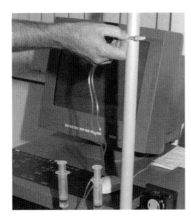

Figure 4.8 Machine correctly calibrated; manometer tube held at 50 cm H$_2$O on the equipment

4.8.3.3 Air-Filled Catheters

Air-filled catheters are checked in the same way as solid-state catheter-tip transducers.

Learning Points

- Pressure can be measured using water-filled, solid-state or air-filled catheters during subtracted cystometry. The use of air-filled catheters during cystometry has not been validated.
- Water-filled lines connected to external pressure transducers are prone to movement artefact.
- Solid-state catheters have a microtransducer in the catheter tip and are not connected to external pressure transducers.
- The Medicine and Healthcare Products Regulatory Agency recommends changing domes, manometry tubing and syringes between patients to prevent cross-infection.
- Calibration of the flowmeter can be checked by using a constant-flow bottle or checking the volume recorded after pouring a known volume into the measuring jug.

- Calibration of the urodynamics machine can be checked by raising tubing ends to a height of 50 cm above atmosphere, marked against a ruler, after zeroing the transducers to atmosphere.
- Transducers are zeroed to atmospheric pressure at the beginning of each test.

References

1. NHS Purchasing and Supply Agency Centre for Evidence-based Purchasing. *Buyers' Guide: Urodynamic Systems.* CEP08045. London; 2008. www.nbt.nhs.uk/sites/default/files/CEP09037.pdf. Accessed December 2009.

2. Gammie A, Clarkson B, Constantinou C, et al. International Continence Society guidelines on urodynamic equipment performance. *Neurourol Urodyn.* 2014;33:370–9.

3. Abrams P, Cardozo L, Fall M, et al. The standardisation of terminology of lower urinary tract function: report from the standardisation sub-committee of the International Continence Society. *Neurourol Urodyn.* 2002;21:167–78.

4. Schäfer W, Abrams P, Liao L, et al. Good urodynamic practices: uroflowmetry, filling cystometry, and pressure-flow studies. *Neurourol Urodyn.* 2002;21:261–74.

5. Rosier PF, Schaefer W, Lose G, et al. International Continence Society Good Urodynamic Practices and Terms 2016: Urodynamics, uroflowmetry, cystometry, and pressure-flow study. *Neurourol Urodyn.* 2017;36:1243–60.

6. Abrams P, Damaser MS, Niblett P, et al. Air filled, including "air-charged," catheters in urodynamic studies: does the evidence justify their use?. *Neurourol Urodyn.* 2017;36:1234–42.

7. Chu A. Dome set-up in urodynamics. *Neurourol Urodyn.* 2007;26:594.

8. Medicines and Healthcare Products Regulatory Agency. *The Reuse of Medical Devices Supplied for Single Use Only.* Device Bulletin DB2006(04). London: Department of Health; 2006. www.mhra.gov.uk/Publications/Safetyguidance/Device Bulletins/CON2024995.

Urodynamic Flow Rate Testing

Laura Thomas, Marcus Drake and Ahmed Shaban

Flow rate testing is a simple, non-invasive test which can provide useful clinical information, although with important limitations. It is an assessment of the volume passed in unit time and is often undertaken in conjunction with other measurements, most notably post-void residual urine volume (PVR) measurement. This chapter covers flow rate testing in females and males but many of the examples relate to conditions found only in men. The principles of interpretation remain the same irrespective of gender.

5.1 The Role of Flow Rate Testing

Many professional urological advisory bodies recommend urine flow rates as a baseline assessment for individuals experiencing lower urinary tract symptoms (LUTS) [1,2]. Given their non-invasive nature, flow rates are a useful tool, both pre- and post-administration of medication, and provide information on patient's urinary stream as well as ability to empty the bladders fully.

5.2 How to Perform a Flow Rate Test

The set-up for uroflowmetry has been described in Chapter 4. The flow machine should be set up in a private area and all efforts should be made to make sure the environment makes the patient as comfortable as possible.

The two most common types of flow meter are:

Gravimetric (weight transducer): the weight of urine voided is measured over time; the flow rate is calculated from the rate of change in weight of urine.

Rotating disc: as the urinary stream falls onto a spinning disc, it increases the weight of the disc, so the motor has to increase power to keep the disc spinning. The flow rate is proportionate to the power needed to keep the disc spinning at the same rate.

Both approaches are widely employed in current commercial systems. They are prone to variations in reliability and need to be calibrated before use. Regular checks are needed at intervals specified by the manufacturer and should also be done if the equipment is moved or disturbed.

5.2.1 Preparation for the Test

Patients should bring with them a completed pre-test frequency volume chart/bladder diary, which will show the patients' typical and maximum voided volume. It is important that the flows recorded are representative of a patient's normal void and therefore the bladder diary is an essential tool to compare with clinical voids; a bladder diary enables comparison of the flow test volume against larger volume voided in day-to-day life. Patients should be well hydrated on arrival and prepared to wait for as long as needed to obtain an adequate result. The patient should be warned that the process can take some time. If they are in a rush to get somewhere else, representative flow rate results will be difficult to obtain.

5.2.2 Performing the Test

Instruct patient a to void normally and in their normal voiding position. Men should aim at one point on the funnel and avoid squeezing the urethra or letting the stream 'wander'. Post-void residual volume (PVR) should ideally be measured within 10 minutes of voiding. The patient may be required to void two to three times due to intra-individual variability, which could affect the conclusions drawn [3]. Adequacy of voided volume should be assessed at the time, referring back to the patient's bladder diary to determine whether it is representative of a normal volume. Voided volumes of over 150 ml are ideal for producing reproducible flow curves [4].

5.3 What Is Assessed and How It Is Interpreted

Several parameters are evaluated with flow rate testing:

Voided volume – the total volume passed via the patient's urethra into the flowmeter.
Maximum flow rate – maximum value on the flow rate, excluding any artefacts.
Voiding time – total time the patient is voiding for.
Flow time – total time there is measurable flow being recorded on the flowmeter.
Time to maximum flow – time between onset of flow and maximum rate of flow.
PVR – volume of urine left in the bladder after voiding (ultrasound or catheter).
Urine flow curve shape – the pattern of flow presented on a graph.

5.3.1 Voided Volume

When combined with the PVR, the volume passed provides information on the storage capacity and is also one of the parameters presented on a flow rate nomogram. Flow rate nomograms clearly show an effect of voided volume on flow rate [5,6]. At low voided volume, Q_{max} may be artefactually reduced. Most clinicians recommend evaluating flow rate only above a voided volume of 150 ml.

Above 550 ml, the bladder starts to overfill, causing artefactual reduction in Q_{max}. Some people can only void at high volumes; this information can be obtained by analysing the frequency volume chart and PVR is often elevated in such individuals.

5.3.2 Maximum Flow Rate

Normal ranges of maximum flow rate (Q_{max}) have been worked out by screening large populations of asymptomatic individuals. They tend to vary based on age and gender. In women, the normal Q_{max} is 20–36 ml/s, increasing by 5.6 ml/s/100 ml voided volume [7].

Q_{max} is affected by voided volume, so nomograms (Liverpool nomograms [5] and Siroky nomograms [6]) have been developed to aid interpretation. Where Q_{max} is significantly below normal (usually taken as two standard deviations below the expected value on a nomogram), there are several possible explanations:

- reduced bladder contractility
- low voided volume
- patient is inhibited (bashful voider)
- equipment has not recorded properly or been calibrated accurately
- bladder outlet obstruction.

5.3.3 Voiding Time and Flow Time

In patients with a 'normal' flow rate and flow pattern, it is likely that the voiding and flow times will be the same. Discrepancies occur when patient's voiding is not continuous and thus produces an intermittent flow curve with periods of non-measureable flow. Patients with terminal dribbling, whose final period of voiding may not meet the threshold for measureable flow, may also exhibit different voiding and flow times.

5.3.4 Urine Flow Rate Curve

The shape of the flow curve provides some hints as to the nature of a person's diagnosis. The normal curve should have a rapid upstroke, a curve with a clear Q_{max} and decline quickly to end cleanly (see Case 5.1 at the end of this chapter). This is often described as 'bell shaped', although the trace is rarely symmetrical.

There are a number of characteristic flow patterns that have been described and although they are not diagnostic, they are often thought to act as an indicators of the individual's underlying pathology. It is, however, key to remember that a description of flow pattern should refer to just the pattern of flow and not the potential cause. Further work is needed to better clarify the terms frequently used, but until then the most common ones are:

Urethral stricture	Rapid upstroke, constant low flow rate giving a 'plateau appearance' and downstroke ends cleanly (see Case 5.1 on page 32).
Fluctuating	Continuous flow with several peaks in Q_{max} often caused by repeated Valsalva manoeuvres such as during straining.
Intermittent	A non-sustained flow rate which stops and starts within the voiding period (see Figure 5.3).
Supervoider	Very high Q_{max} and rapid upstroke and downstroke. Not diagnostic, but people with detrusor overactivity generally have flow rates at the top end of the range (see Case 5.4) [8].
Artefacts	Overestimates of Q_{max} owing to a high-speed squirt of urine from release of compression (Figure 5.1) or the stream 'wandering' on the spinning disc (Figure 5.2). Kicking or knocking the flow meter will also produce an artefactual spike in flow rate.

Attempts to measure objective parameters for describing flow patterns have been made [5].

5.4 Nomograms

The majority of work conducted around urine flow rates had focused on their ability to predict bladder outlet obstruction in men. Less attention has been paid to their role in females and children; however, with the introduction of female continence surgery, there is a greater possibility of female outlet obstruction, and therefore further attention may need to be directed towards this.

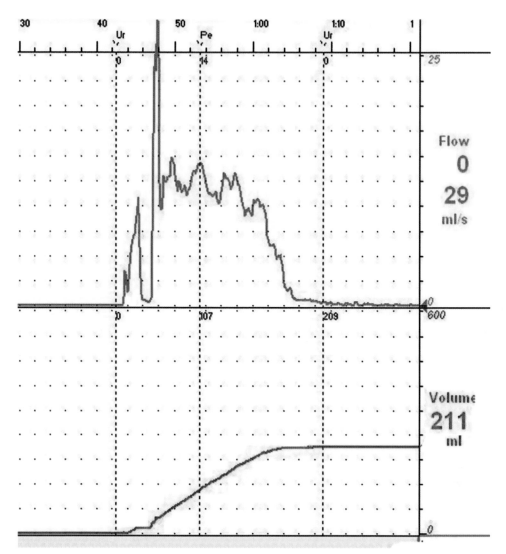

Figure 5.1 A common flow rate artefact in men with lower urinary tract symptoms. Shortly after start of voiding, the tip of the urethra has been held shut to build up pressure. Release then causes a sudden spurt, before the true voiding pattern re-establishes. The flow meter has recorded Q_{max} as 29 ml/s but examination of the trace quickly shows the artefactual nature of the recorded maximum and that the true value is near 13 ml/s

Nomograms display the relationship between two variables, most commonly voided or bladder volume and maximum flow rate. They are not able to provide a precise diagnosis but instead display a predictive statistical model which exhibits the probability of normal flow. There are a number of different nomograms used across clinics with variable adjustments made for demographics such as age and gender [6,9]. The Liverpool Nomograms [5] are also a well-known tool used in many centres which, like Kadow et al. [9], use voided rather than bladder volume and have both male and female graphs. It is evident that

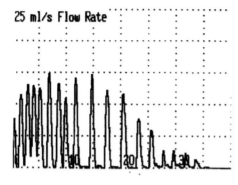

Figure 5.2 Intermittent stream resulting from a man allowing his urinary stream to wander over the collecting funnel; the voided volume was small and the trace unrepresentative

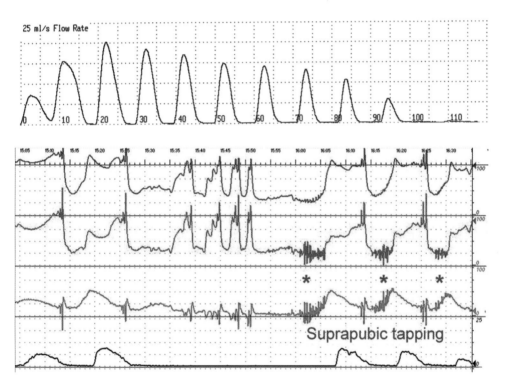

Figure 5.3 A young man with partial lumbar spinal cord injury. Top panel shows a highly interrupted flow pattern. In the lower panel, subsequent cystometry showed straining. The blue asterisks (labelled 'suprapubic tapping') show three occasions when the patient used banging on the suprapubic area to elicit a bladder contraction, causing expulsion of a little more urine each time

most of the well-known nomograms are based on male patients and provide guidance on the interpretation of male flow rates only. On the whole, interpretation of female flows is made more difficult by the lack of definite reference values for uroflow parameters in women and as such further research into flow rates in normal women may be warranted [10]. The sensitivity of a flow rate test has been shown to increase when the whole bladder volume is considered rather than voided volume alone, providing guidance on potential advances in future nomograms [11].

(a)

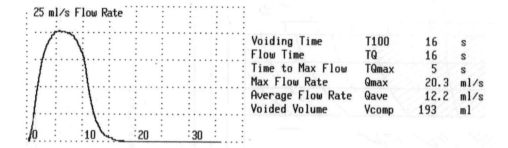

Voiding Time	T100	16	s
Flow Time	TQ	16	s
Time to Max Flow	TQmax	5	s
Max Flow Rate	Qmax	20.3	ml/s
Average Flow Rate	Qave	12.2	ml/s
Voided Volume	Vcomp	193	ml

(b)

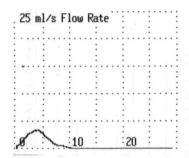

Voiding Time	T100	9	s
Flow Time	TQ	9	s
Time to Max Flow	TQmax	3	s
Max Flow Rate	Qmax	3.4	ml/s
Average Flow Rate	Qave	1.9	ml/s
Voided Volume	Vcomp	17	ml

(c)

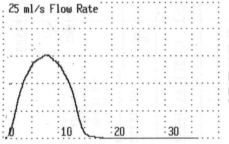

Voiding Time	T100	16	s
Flow Time	TQ	16	s
Time to Max Flow	TQmax	7	
Max Flow Rate	Qmax	15.2	ml/s
Average Flow Rate	Qave	9.5	ml/s
Voided Volume	Vcomp	149	ml

Figure 5.4 Uroflowmetry traces showing: (a) a normal flow rate; (b) and (c) that voided volume has a substantial effect on Q_{max} (Case 5.1)

5.5 Women with Incontinence

Low Q_{max} may be associated with voiding dysfunction after continence surgery or pelvic organ prolapse. A high PVR may occur infrequently after anticholinergic drug administration in overactive bladder syndrome.

5.6 Men with Voiding Symptoms

A low Q_{max} is not diagnostic for bladder outlet obstruction but it is a guide for the success of treatment, and regular flow rate testing during follow-up can be a guide to recurrence (see Case 5.1).

5.7 Patients with Neurological Disease

Interpretation is complicated by the greater range of possible pathologies. Suprapubic 'tapping' (banging the hand on to the suprapubic area, the shock of which can set off a short-lived bladder contraction, leading to partial emptying) is typically combined with straining (Figure 5.3).

Low Q_{max} can also result from bladder outlet obstruction, with failure of relaxation of bladder neck, detrusor sphincter dyssynergia and outlet distortion (as in pelvic organ prolapse) possibilities, in addition to stricture or benign prostate enlargement.

Elevated PVR can occur in conjunction with detrusor failure or bladder outlet obstruction.

5.8 Clinical Cases

Four cases are presented, with the first two cases in male patients with voiding obstruction. Those cases have been included as the physical principles with regard to flow are applicable to both genders even though clinical conditions will differ.

Case 5.1

A 70-year-old male with slight enlargement of prostate gland on clinical examination (Figure 5.4).

Three uroflowmetry traces with different voided volumes are shown. Figure 5.4a shows a normal flow rate, with a rapid upstroke, good Q_{max} and slightly less rapid downstroke. In this man, there is only a low probability of bladder outlet obstruction. Three flows have been recorded for the same patient, with the top (Figure 5.4a) being entirely normal; the middle (Figure 5.4b) and lower traces (Figure 5.4c) show that voided volume has a substantial effect on Q_{max} and a reduction in Q_{max} can arise when voided volume is inadequate, even in the absence of bladder outlet obstruction.

Case 5.2

A male with a history of voiding difficulty presenting in acute urinary retention (Figure 5.5).

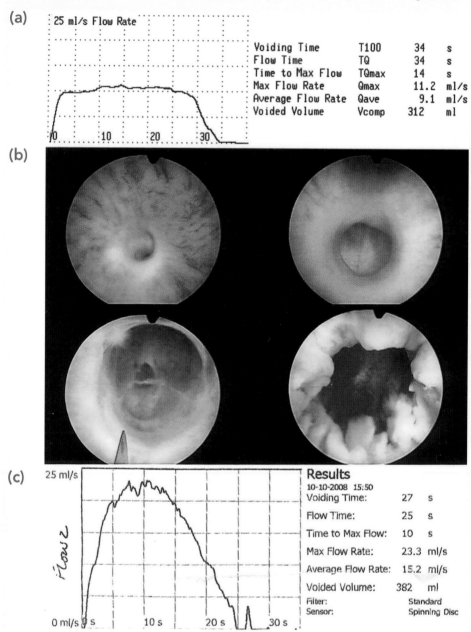

(a)

25 ml/s Flow Rate			
Voiding Time	T100	34	s
Flow Time	TQ	34	s
Time to Max Flow	TQmax	14	s
Max Flow Rate	Qmax	11.2	ml/s
Average Flow Rate	Qave	9.1	ml/s
Voided Volume	Vcomp	312	ml

(b)

(c)

25 ml/s

flow

0 ml/s 0 s   10 s   20 s   30 s

Results

10-10-2008 15:50

Voiding Time:	27	s
Flow Time:	25	s
Time to Max Flow:	10	s
Max Flow Rate:	23.3	ml/s
Average Flow Rate:	15.2	ml/s
Voided Volume:	382	ml
Filter:	Standard	
Sensor:	Spinning Disc	

Figure 5.5 Voiding difficulty: (a) cystometry showing stricture pattern flow rate; (b) stages in urethrotomy, starting with the initial view of a tight stricture, with increasing depth of urethrotomy, culminating in the final view seen in the bottom right picture; (c) flow rate pattern showing that urethrotomy has achieved a normal trace (Case 5.2)

Figure 5.5a shows voiding cystometry with stricture pattern flow rate, illustrating a normal upstroke, a plateau with reduced Q_{max} and a normal downstroke. This series also illustrates the use of flow rate testing to evaluate surgical outcome. The endoscopic pictures (Figure 5.5b) show stages in this man's urethrotomy, starting with the initial view of a tight stricture, with increasing depth of urethrotomy culminating in the final view seen in the bottom right endoscopic picture. The depth of scarring was severe, such that scarring is clearly apparent till the end of the operation, and recurrence appears a distinct possibility. The flow rate pattern in Figure 5.5c shows that urethrotomy has achieved a normal trace. Flow rate testing will be a valuable means of assessing recurrence during subsequent follow-up.

Case 5.3

A 58-year-old female complaining of vaginal prolapse, slow intermittent urinary stream and recurrent urinary tract infections. Previous history of colposuspension (Figure 5.6).

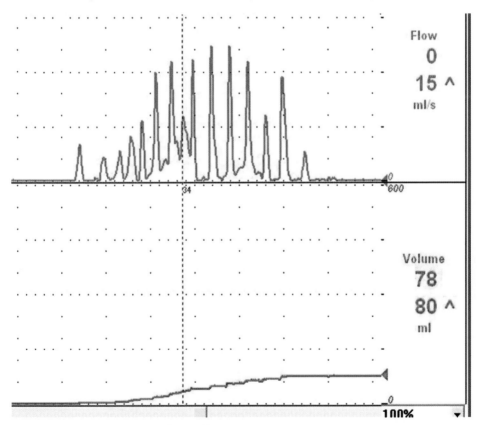

Figure 5.6 Severe straining pattern (Case 5.3)

The uroflowmetry shows an interrupted flow with several peaks in flow rate indicative of severe abdominal straining. A residual 250 ml was drained with the filling catheter at onset of cystometry. Voiding cystometry confirmed a diagnosis of abdominal straining due to obstructive voiding, secondary to previous surgery and large enterocele.

Case 5.4

A 52-year-old female with a history of frequency, urgency and occasional urge incontinence. No voiding difficulties (Figure 5.7).

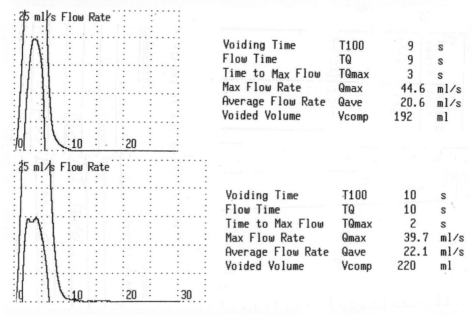

Voiding Time	T100	9	s
Flow Time	TQ	9	s
Time to Max Flow	TQmax	3	s
Max Flow Rate	Qmax	44.6	ml/s
Average Flow Rate	Qave	20.6	ml/s
Voided Volume	Vcomp	192	ml

Voiding Time	T100	10	s
Flow Time	TQ	10	s
Time to Max Flow	TQmax	2	s
Max Flow Rate	Qmax	39.7	ml/s
Average Flow Rate	Qave	22.1	ml/s
Voided Volume	Vcomp	220	ml

Figure 5.7 Uroflowmetry showing a 'super voider' (Case 5.4)

The uroflowmetry shows a very rapid upstroke and downstroke with very high Q_{max}. This 'supervoider' was subsequently shown to have detrusor overactivity urodynamically.

Learning Points

- There are two common types of flow rate systems: gravimetric and rotating disc.
- Information on typical and maximum voided volumes can be obtained from the pre-test frequency volume chart.
- Intra-individual variation in flow rate may necessitate performing two or three voids.
- Most clinicians assess flow rate when the voided volume exceeds 150 ml because of the risk of artefact at lower voided volumes.
- Normal flow has a rapid upstroke and a 'bell-shaped' curve.
- A plateau-shaped flow pattern is observed in the presence of a urethral stricture.
- A residual of less than 100 ml is not regarded as clinically significant in asymptomatic patients.

References

1. The National Institute For Health and Care Excellence (NICE). Lower urinary tract symptoms in men: management. 2015 Update. www.nice.org.uk/guidance/cg97

2. European Association of Urology (EAU) Non-neurogenic Male LUTS Guideline. 2017. http://uroweb.org/wp-content/uploads/13-Non-Neurogenic-MaleLUTS_2017_web.pdf

3. Matzkin H, van der Zwaag R, Chen Y, et al. How reliable is a single measurement of urinary flow in the diagnosis of obstruction in benign prostatic hyperplasia? *Br J Urol.* 1993;72:181–6.

4. Schäfer W, Abrams P, Liao L, et al. Good urodynamic practices: uroflowmetry, filling cystometry, and pressure-flow studies. *Neurourol Urodyn.* 2002;21: 261–74.

5. Haylen BT, Ashby D, Sutherst JR, Frazer MI, West CR. Maximum and average urine flow rates in normal male and female populations – the Liverpool nomograms. *Br J Urol.* 1989;64:30–8.

6. Siroky MB, Olsson CA, Krane RJ. The flow rate nomogram: I. Development. *J Urol.* 1979;122:665–8.

7. Jorgensen JB, Colstrup H, Frimodt-Moller C. Uroflow in women: an overview and suggestions for the future. *Int Urogynecol J Pelvic Floor Dysfunct.* 1998;9:33–6.

8. Haylen BT, Parys BT, Anyaegbunam WI, Ashby D, West CR. Urine flow rates in male and female urodynamic patients compared with the Liverpool nomograms. *Br J Urol.* 1990;65:483–7.

9. Kadow C, Howells S, Lewis P, Abrams P. A flow rate nomogram for normal males over the age of 50. Proceedings of the 15th Annual Meeting of the International Continence Society, London, 1985:138–9.

10. Sorel MR, Reitsma HJB, Rosier PFWM, Bosch RJLHR, de Kort LMO Uroflowmetry in healthy women: a systematic review. *Neurourol Urodyn,* 2017;36:953–9.

11. Al-Hayek S, Belal M, Abrams P. How reliable is non-invasive uroflowmetry in predicting the presence of bladder outlet obstruction in men? *J Urol.* 2006;175:437.

Chapter

6

The Cystometrogram[*]

Angie Rantell

6.1 Introduction

According to the International Continence Society (ICS) (2016), cystometry is the continuous fluid filling of the bladder via a transurethral catheter (or other route, e.g. suprapubic or mitrofanoff), with at least intravesical and abdominal pressure measurements and display of detrusor pressure, including cough (stress) testing. Cystometry ends with 'permission to void' or with incontinence of the total bladder content [1].

Details of setting up the equipment for cystometry are described in Chapter 4. Generic standards for subtracted dual-channel cystometry can be found in the *Joint Statement on Minimum Standards for Urodynamic Practice in the UK* [2]. For good practice in cystometry, the fluid type, temperature, filling method and rate, catheter size, pressure-recording technique and patient position should all be specified, and these will be discussed in this chapter.

6.2 Prior to Conducting Cystometry

6.2.1 Residual Urine

Post-void residual (PVR) urine is assessed immediately prior to cystometry (usually following uroflowmetry – see Chapters 4 and 5) by a dedicated bladder scanner, conventional ultrasound scanner or via inserting and draining the residual urine through the urethral filling catheter.

The recommendation of draining the PVR urine before cystometry is controversial and many investigators choose to perform the cystometrogram on top of any PVR [3].

6.2.2 Checking for Urinary Tract Infection (UTI)

Cystometry is usually postponed if the patient has a urinary tract infection (UTI) because this could influence the urodynamic findings. A symptomatic UTI may lead to increased bladder sensation and reduced cystometric capacity, and cause urinary incontinence in patients who do not normally experience these symptoms.

Testing a specimen of urine with reagent strips for nitrites and leucocytes can provide a reasonable screening tool in the urodynamics clinic, with a sensitivity of at least 96.4% and a specificity of at least 88.5% [4]. If nitrites and leucocytes are present, there is a strong possibility of a UTI and the cystometrogram should not be carried out. A specimen of urine

---

[*] Updated from original chapter by Gordon Hosker and Joanne Townsend.

Table 6.1 International Continence Society recommendations for baseline pressures at onset of filling cystometry

	Pressure (cm H_2O)	
	Minimum	**Maximum**
p_{ves}	5	50
p_{abd}	5	50
p_{det}	−5	15

should be sent for microscopy and any infection should be appropriately treated. If a significant residual urine is noted, this should be managed appropriately.

6.3 Starting the Test

Pressure-recording techniques and catheter selection methods are discussed in detail in Chapter 4. The pressure catheters are prepared and inserted using an aseptic technique. The agreed reference height for external transducers is the level of the superior border of the symphysis pubis [5].

6.3.1 Initial Pressures – Resting Intravesical and Abdominal Pressures

Gentle flushing of both catheter channels should be performed to ensure that the catheters are not kinked or that the catheter holes are not blocked or in contact with the bladder wall prior to establishing initial resting pressures.

The values for abdominal pressure (p_{abd}), intravesical pressure (p_{ves}) and detrusor pressure (p_{det}) should be compared with the values shown in Table 6.1. The values of p_{abd} and p_{ves} will be at the lower end of the range if the patient is small and lying down and at the higher end of the range if the patient is large and standing up. If the values are outside these ranges, then:

- recheck the set-up before starting to fill;
- ensure that the external transducers are positioned at the upper level of the symphysis pubis;
- zero external transducers to atmospheric pressure;
- check that the pressure lines have not slipped out of position (expelled catheter); and
- ensure that the patient is not faecally loaded.

If the problem persists, proceed with the cystometrogram only if you consider that you have a valid explanation for the baseline pressures being outside the expected range.

6.3.2 Checking for Artefacts

Before commencing filling, ask the patient to cough to check that the pressure lines are recording intravesical and abdominal pressures correctly. Ideally, the strength of the cough should induce a pressure increase of about 100 cm H_2O. When the patient coughs, there should be an equal acute rise in both the abdominal and intravesical pressure traces. The detrusor pressure trace, which is derived by subtracting the abdominal pressure trace from the intravesical pressure trace, should show little movement (Figure 6.1) [3].

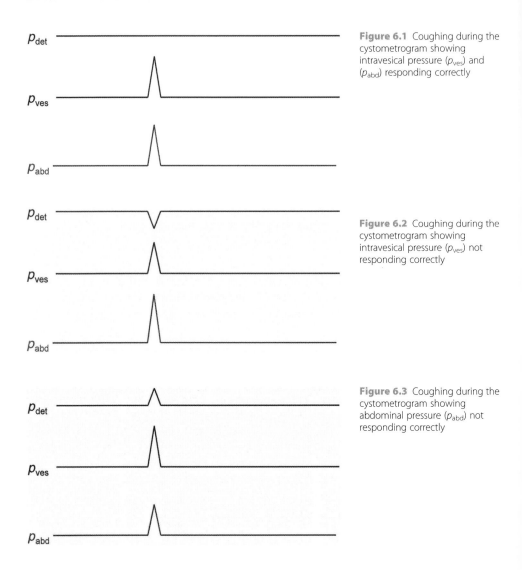

Figure 6.1 Coughing during the cystometrogram showing intravesical pressure (p_{ves}) and (p_{abd}) responding correctly

Figure 6.2 Coughing during the cystometrogram showing intravesical pressure (p_{ves}) not responding correctly

Figure 6.3 Coughing during the cystometrogram showing abdominal pressure (p_{abd}) not responding correctly

If the rise in intravesical pressure is smaller than the rise in abdominal pressure (Figure 6.2), this indicates a problem with the intravesical pressure recording (see Chapter 9).

If the rise in intravesical pressure is greater than the rise in abdominal pressure (Figure 6.3), this indicates a problem with the abdominal pressure recording (see Chapter 9).

ICS 2016 describes common artefacts that may occur when setting up cystometry. These include:

Dead signal – a signal that does not show small pressure fluctuations and does not adequately respond to patient straining, movement or coughing.

Pressure drift – continuous, slow fall or rise in pressure that is physiologically inexplicable.

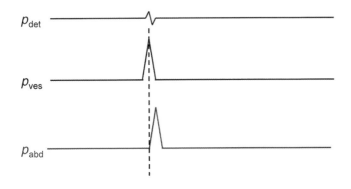

Figure 6.4 Biphasic artefact in detrusor pressure (p_{det}) arising from timing differences between the recording of intravesical pressure (p_{ves}) and detrusor pressure (p_{abd})

Poor pressure transmission – that occurs when the cough/effort pressure peaks of the p_{ves} and p_{abd} are not nearly equal.

A biphasic artefact on coughing in p_{det} (Figure 6.4) is caused by small physical differences in the two pressure lines that cause their respective transducers to respond at slightly different times to the impulse of the cough. Provided that the amplitude of the pressure rises in p_{abd} and p_{ves} is equivalent, correction is not required and the next phase of the cystometrogram can be directly carried out.

6.3.3 Selecting the Filling Rate

There is a lack of evidence relating to the optimum filling rate. For a neurologically intact adult, current ICS recommendations report that filling rate should be standardised on each individual patient's typical voided volumes (including an estimation of the PVR value) to prevent too fast filling [1]. A filling rate in ml/min of roughly 10% of the largest voided volume at a constant rate is recommended. For example, if the maximum functional capacity is 500 ml, a filling rate of 50 ml/min is recommended. The initial filling rate may vary between 30 and 100 ml/min.

For neurological patients or if marked detrusor overactivity is suspected, select a less provocative rate, such as 10 ml/min [3]. This gives a better chance of achieving a voiding study at the end of filling cystometry. In paediatrics, the filling rate is calculated based on the child's age and weight.

6.3.4 Temperature of the Filling Medium

Usually 0.9% physiological saline is used (except in video urodynamics when a radio-opaque dye will be used). Low temperatures can artefactually induce detrusor overactivity, particularly at low bladder volumes. There is no evidence to show that body temperature should be preferred to room temperature. Make sure that the fluid has actually achieved at least normal room temperature (20°C) before instilling it into the patient [4].

6.3.5 Patient Position

Position can influence the outcome of cystometry [6]. It is recommended that cystometry be performed in the vertical position (standing or normally seated) whenever physically possible. The position adopted at the start of cystometry can be dependent on the degree of mobility of the patient.

Box 6.1 Patient sensations as defined by the International Continence Society [6]

Sensation	Definition
First sensation of filling (FSF)	The feeling the patient has during filling cystometry, when she first becomes aware of bladder filling
First desire to void (FDV)	The feeling, during filling cystometry, that would lead the patient to pass urine at the next convenient moment, but voiding can be delayed if necessary
Strong desire to void (SDV)	The feeling, during filling cystometry, of a persistent desire to void without the fear of leakage
Maximum cystometric capacity (MCC)	The volume at which the patient feels that her capacity (MCC) can no longer delay micturition (i.e. has a strong desire to void)
Urgency	A sudden compelling desire to void during the cystometrogram (which should be recorded on the cystometrogram and noted if it reproduces the symptoms)

6.4 The Cystometrogram

While bladder filling is occurring, the pressures are observed on the cystometrogram. All patient sensations should be annotated on the cystometrogram. Sensation may be classified as normal, increased, reduced or absent. The complaint of pain during cystometry is abnormal, and if reported, the site, character and duration should be noted. The bladder diary provides a good idea of the patient's normal functional bladder capacity and is helpful in conducting the cystometrogram [5]. The International Continence Society has defined some of the sensations (Box 6.1) [7].

During filling, the patient should be asked to cough every minute (Figure 6.5). If good subtraction is lost, the test should be stopped and the lines checked (see Chapter 9). If the patient is set over a flowmeter during cystometry, leakage will be recorded on the flow trace. If the urgency subsides, the operator may wish to continue filling, perhaps at a slower speed, depending on how much fluid is required in the bladder.

6.5 Normal Detrusor Function

When detrusor function is normal, there is little or no change or contraction in p_{det} during bladder filling despite provocation (Figure 6.6). Table 6.2 shows some of the parameters of filling cystometry in a series of 72 women without any urinary dysfunction. This study suggests that the range of normal maximum cystometric capacity is large and varies between 360 and 800 ml.

Bladder compliance is the relationship between change in volume in the bladder and change in pressure. Usually, compliance is calculated from the change in detrusor pressure from an empty bladder up to the cystometric capacity. Therefore, it can be seen from the cystometrogram in Figure 6.6 that p_{det} has risen from 0 to 4 cm H_2O as the bladder fills to 550 ml, which gives a compliance of 138 ml/cm H_2O.

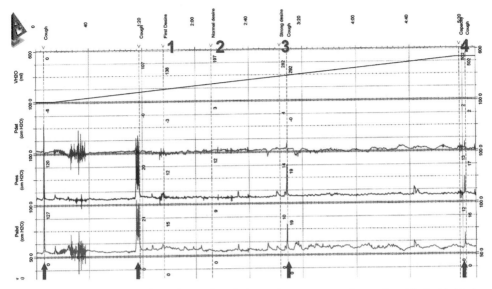

Figure 6.5 Cystometrogram with regular coughing (red arrows) to assess recording quality while the bladder is being filled at 100 ml/min. The operator has recorded when the patient has a first desire to void (1), a normal desire to void (2), a strong desire to void (3) and maximum cystometric capacity (4)

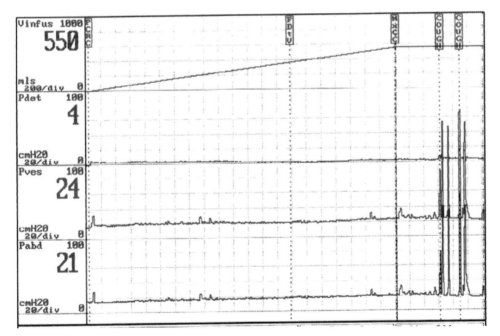

Figure 6.6 A normal filling cystometrogram

Table 6.2 Cystometric parameters in asymptomatic women (*n* = 72) during filling cystometry; filled with 0.9% physiological saline at body temperature at a rate of 100 ml/min

Parameter	Mean	SD	Minimum	Maximum
Age (years)	41.4	10.1	25	75
Parity	2.3	1.6	0	7
Residual urine (ml)	11	13	0	60
First desire to void (ml)	304	116	60	640
Maximum cystometric capacity (ml)	543	94	360	800
Compliance (ml/cm H_2O)	124	150	31	800

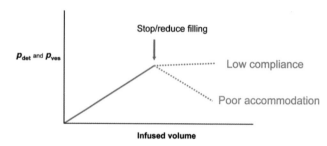

Figure 6.7 The difference between low compliance and 'poor accommodation'

6.6 Abnormal Detrusor Function

6.6.1 Low (Poor) Compliance

Some bladders are 'stiffer' than others and do not have the same elasticity as normal bladders; for example, radiotherapy in the region of the bladder causes stiffening or a large pelvic mass pressing on the bladder (fibroid uterus). Urodynamically, this manifests itself as a steep rise in detrusor (and intravesical) pressure during filling.

Typically, the value of compliance is less than 30 ml/cm H_2O and often associated with a reduced capacity. However, before a diagnosis of low compliance is made, filling is stopped. If the detrusor pressure remains abnormally high, the bladder is of low compliance. If the detrusor pressure drops to normal values when filling is stopped, then this is not low compliance but might be termed poor accommodation (Figure 6.7), as some bladders need time to accommodate fluid filling them at non-physiological rates.

6.6.2 High Compliance

'High compliance' describes a large capacity 'floppy' bladder. Generally speaking, there is an underlying neurological cause. Typically, the value of compliance is considerably greater than 100 ml/cm H_2O and capacities of more than 1 l are not uncommon.

6.6.3 Detrusor Overactivity

Detrusor overactivity describes the involuntary detrusor contractions occurring during the filling phase of cystometry, which may be spontaneous or provoked. Phasic detrusor

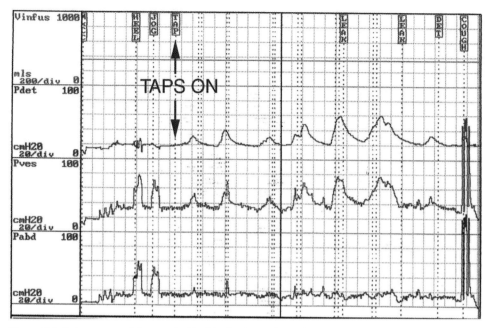

Figure 6.8 Detrusor overactivity provoked by listening to running water

overactivity consists of waves of detrusor contractions seen during filling, which may or may not be associated with incontinence. Terminal detrusor overactivity is a single involuntary detrusor contraction occurring at cystometric capacity, which cannot be suppressed and results in incontinence, usually resulting in bladder emptying [7].

There is no lower limit to the amplitude of an involuntary detrusor contraction but high quality urodynamic technique is imperative to be able to interpret low-pressure waves (less than 5 cm H_2O) correctly.

According to the ICS/IUGA joint terminology report (2010) [8] symptoms, for example, urgency and/or urgency incontinence may or may not occur.

6.6.4 Patient Position, Provocative Manoeuvres and Detrusor Overactivity

If no detrusor overactivity is seen in the supine position, the patient should either sit down or stand up at cystometric capacity. The overactivity may only be seen if the patient is in a position other than supine. (Remember to relocate the transducers at the level of the symphysis pubis if the patient changes her position with fluid-filled lines [6].)

Other provocative manoeuvres to demonstrate or confirm the absence of detrusor overactivity include heel bouncing, jogging on the spot, listening to running water (Figure 6.8), washing hands under running water, coughing and refilling the bladder in a different position.

6.7 Urodynamic Stress Incontinence

ICS/IUGA defines urodynamic stress incontinence as the involuntary leakage of urine seen during filling cystometry, associated with a raised abdominal pressure but in the absence of a detrusor contraction [8]. Leakage seen during coughing while the cystometric trace shows no evidence of a detrusor contraction confirms the diagnosis.

Coughing to demonstrate or confirm the absence of urodynamic stress incontinence is best performed with the patient standing or sitting on the commode. Other factors that induce the patient's symptoms, such as walking on the spot or shouting, may be employed to reproduce the reported symptoms.

If a separate filling line is used, then it should generally be removed before testing for urodynamic stress incontinence. Additionally, any prolapse should be gently supported, for example, by a pessary, the blade of a speculum or a finger, and the patient asked to cough again to assess for occult stress incontinence.

6.8 At the End of Filling Cystometry

It is usual to proceed to the voiding phase of urodynamics at this point. When the catheters are removed at the end of the voiding phase, patients should be warned that they might experience some stinging during subsequent micturition. This sensation is common and usually lasts for a few hours and will resolve. Advising patients to drink plenty of fluids may help to reduce the risk of developing a UTI. However, if these irritative symptoms persist for more than 48 hours, the patient should be instructed to take a specimen of urine to their general practitioner to check for a UTI [9].

6.9 The Urodynamics Environment

The clinical environment in which urodynamic tests are performed can have a significant impact on the quality of the test and patient experience. The clinical area should have a room with adequate space to fit all the clinical equipment and consumables, have separate toilet and changing facilities and a suitable waiting area with access to drinking water. The environment should be designed to ensure patients are as comfortable as possible and to relieve anxiety as well as maintaining their privacy and dignity. Patients who are very anxious or feeling cold may experience shivering that will produce an artefact on the traces, reduce the quality of the test and potentially impact upon bladder sensations and pain levels. The environment should also have appropriate facilities for monitoring vital signs or cardiopulmonary resuscitation as there is the potential for patients to experience vasovagal attack during the test due to pain or anxiety.

6.10 Clinical Cases

Case 6.1

A 59-year-old woman with a history of radical hysterectomy and adjuvant radiotherapy for Stage 2a cervical carcinoma (Figure 6.9).

She complains of symptoms of urinary frequency, nocturia, urgency, urgency urinary incontinence and mild stress urinary incontinence. Bladder diary indicates hourly voiding with average voided volumes of 100 ml and maximum volume of 200 ml. No history of urinary tract infection. Filling has been stopped twice during the cystometrogram, and on both of these occasions, as well as at cystometric capacity, the pressure has remained abnormally high, confirming low compliance. The maximum cystometric capacity is 218 ml and the detrusor pressure has risen to a value of about 65 cm H_2O, giving a compliance of 3.4 ml/cm H_2O.

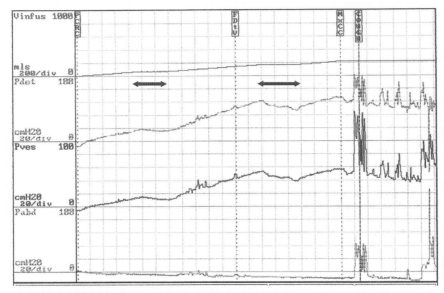

Figure 6.9 Cystometrogram demonstrating low compliance

Case 6.2

Two patients, each with overactive bladder symptoms (Figures 6.10 and 6.11).

In Figure 6.10, when urgency was labelled, there were rises in the red p_{det} trace. The rises were also seen in the purple p_{ves} trace, and hence the evidence of detrusor overactivity.

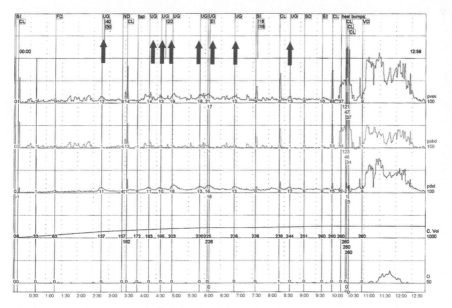

Figure 6.10 Cystometrogram with episodes of urgency labelled

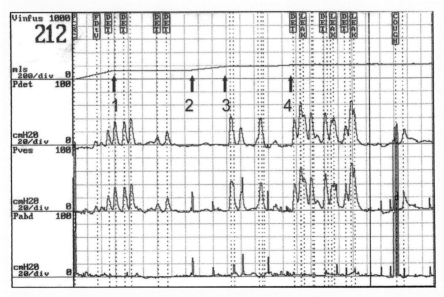

Figure 6.11 Reducing the filling rate when there is marked detrusor overactivity

In Figure 6.11, marked detrusor overactivity is easily demonstrated on initial filling at 100 ml/min. To ensure that sufficient fluid is in the bladder to study voiding, bladder filling is stopped at arrow 1, recommenced at a rate of 30 ml/min at arrow 2, slowed further to 10 ml/min at arrow 3 before stopping filling at arrow 4 (at a reduced capacity of 212 ml).

Case 6.3

A 53-year-old woman with symptoms of leakage of urine on coughing and sneezing. No urinary frequency, urgency or urgency urinary incontinence. No previous surgery (Figure 6.12).

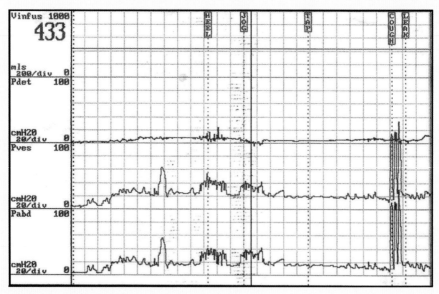

Figure 6.12 Urodynamic stress incontinence

Figure 6.12 shows a bladder which has a maximum cystometric capacity of 433 ml. It is stable throughout heel bouncing, jogging on the spot and listening to running water. The patient then coughs, which produces a strong increase in p_{abd} (red trace); this impinges on the bladder (p_{ves} – blue trace); there is no overactivity seen at this time (p_{det} – purple trace) but urinary leakage is observed: the patient has urodynamic stress incontinence.

Case 6.4

A 47-year-old woman with symptoms of frequency, mild urgency, occasional urgency urinary incontinence and stress urinary incontinence with coughing and bending (Figure 6.13).

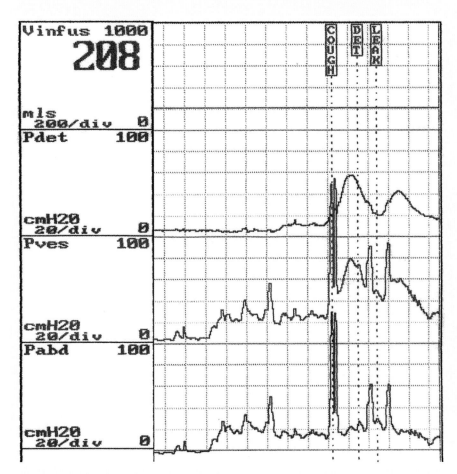

Figure 6.13 Cough-provoked detrusor overactivity

At a cystometric capacity of 208 ml, the patient coughs, which produces a strong increase in p_{abd} (red trace); this impinges on the bladder (p_{ves} – blue trace) and provokes a detrusor contraction (p_{det} – purple trace and p_{ves} – blue trace) and urinary leakage is observed: the patient has cough-provoked detrusor overactivity.

Learning Points

- Cystometry is usually deferred if the patient has a urinary tract infection.
- Initial resting abdominal, intravesical and detrusor pressures should be within the normal range before commencing filling.
- Cough testing should cause an acute and equal rise in abdominal and intravesical pressures with little rise in detrusor pressure.
- Initial filling rate in a non-neurological patient is dependent on maximum functional capacity of 30–100 ml/min.
- The filling medium should be at room temperature (20°C) before filling.
- Cough tests should be performed every minute during filling.
- Low compliance is typically less than 30 ml/cm H_2O and associated with low capacity.
- Detrusor overactivity is not defined by amplitude of detrusor contraction and it may or may not be accompanied by symptoms of urgency or urgency incontinence.
- Urodynamic stress incontinence is the presence of leakage of urine with a rise in intra-abdominal pressure in the absence of a detrusor contraction.
- Provocative testing, such as a change of position or listening to running water, should be used to elicit detrusor overactivity.
- As far as possible, the test should aim to reproduce the patient's symptoms.
- It is important to note that the colours of the pressure lines on the cystometrogram and values displayed will vary between departments and machines, so it is essential to orientate yourself with the format on each cystometrogram before making a diagnosis.

References

1. Rosier PF, Schaefer W, Lose G, et al. International Continence Society Good Urodynamic Practices and Terms 2016: urodynamics, uroflowmetry, cystometry, and pressure-flow study. *Neurourol Urodyn.* 20162017;36(5):1243–60.

2. Working Group of the United Kingdom Continence Society, Abrams P, Eustice S, Gammie A, et al. United Kingdom Continence Society: Minimum standards for urodynamic studies, 2018. *Neurourol Urodyn.* 2019. doi:10.1002/nau.23909. Epub ahead of print.

3. Abrams P. *Urodynamics.* 3rd ed. London: Springer-Verlag; 2006.

4. Preston A, O'Donnell T, Phillips CA. Screening for urinary tract infections in a gynaecological setting: validity and cost-effectiveness of reagent strips. *Br J Biomed Sci.* 1999;56:253–7.

5. Schafer W, Abrams P, Liao L, et al. Good urodynamic practices: uroflowmetry, filling cystometry, and pressure-flow studies. *Neurourol Urodyn.* 2002;21:261–74.

6. Al-Hayek S, Belal M, Abrams P. Does the patient's position influence the detection of detrusor overactivity? *Neurourol Urodyn.* 2008;27:279–86.

7. Abrams P, Cardozo L, Fall M, et al. The standardisation of terminology of lower urinary tract function: report from the Standardisation Sub-committee of the International Continence Society. *Neurourol Urodyn.* 2002;21:167–78.

8. Haylen BT, de Ridder D, Freeman RM, et al. IUGA/ICS joint report on the terminology for female pelvic floor dysfunction. *Neurourol Urodyn.* 2010;29 (1):4–20.

9. Bombieri L, Dance DA, Rienhardt GW, Waterfield A, Freeman RM. Urinary tract infection after urodynamic studies in women: incidence and natural history. *BJU Int.* 1999;83:392–5.

Videocystourethrography

Smita Rajshekhar and Sushma Srikrishna

7.1 Introduction

Videocystourethrography (VCU), also known as videourodynamics, comprises synchronous radiological screening of the urinary tract during subtracted dual-channel filling and voiding cystometry [1].

VCU offers a comprehensive evaluation of the lower urinary tract by combining both anatomical and functional assessments.

7.2 Technical Requirements for VCU

The equipment for dual-channel subtracted cystometry during VCU is identical to that for conventional cystometry described in Chapters 4 and 5. In addition, special equipment – which includes a radio-opaque filling medium and facilities for imaging of the urinary tract – is required. VCU is usually performed within a fluoroscopy unit with a high-resolution image intensifier and a tilt table designed for urodynamics so that the patient can be moved from supine to upright positions during provocative testing and when voiding (Figure 7.1). The professional undertaking VCU should also have completed ionising radiation protection training.

7.3 Conducting VCU

The equipment for subtracted dual-channel cystometry should be set up as described in Chapter 4. Uroflowmetry, insertion of catheters and measurement of residual urine are undertaken in the supine position similar to conventional urodynamics. A nonionic, low osmolality, iodinated contrast medium like iohexol (Omnipaque 140, GE Healthcare) is used to fill the bladder instead of physiological (0.9%) saline. X-ray screening is undertaken as screen shots at intervals during the test rather than continuously, to minimise the patient's exposure to ionising radiation. Most units have a radiographer to perform screening under instruction by the urodynamicist. It would be usual to take images during filling when a patient complains of leakage, at rest in standing position, on provocation during coughs or running taps, during voiding and on completion of voiding. A patient may be asked to interrupt the flow after normal flow is established to allow measurement of p_{iso} or isovolumetric detrusor pressure and to facilitate visualisation of vesicoureteric reflux during simultaneous imaging of the urinary tract.

7.4 Observations during VCU

Real-time imaging of the urinary tract at appropriate stages of filling and voiding cystometry can provide useful additional information to be acquired at each step of the procedure.

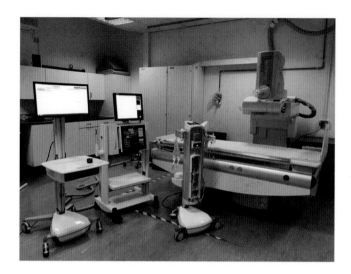

Figure 7.1 Fluoroscopy unit with a high-resolution image intensifier and a tilt table

1. Imaging during filling cystometry: Full bladder at rest – allows morphological assessment of bladder, presence of trabeculations, diverticula, vesicoureteric reflux and any pelvic masses indenting the bladder.
2. Imaging during straining or coughing: Presence and severity of incontinence (in the authors' practice, leaking with the first cough is graded as severe incontinence, leaking during a series of three coughs as moderate leakage and leakage occurring only at the end of five coughs as mild incontinence), evidence of pelvic organ prolapse, and/or bladder neck descent and rotation.
3. Imaging during voiding cystometry: Urethral obstruction or narrowing, dilatation and urethral diverticulum can be noted. Imaging during a 'Stop Test' assesses the voluntary urethral closure mechanism or $p_{\text{det iso}}$ (peak isometric detrusor pressure). A rise in pressure or $p_{\text{det iso}}$ indicates at least some degree of contractility of the detrusor. It also may be used to demonstrate the presence and severity of vesicoureteric reflux. Vesicoureteric reflux can be graded according to the height of reflux up the ureters and degree of dilatation of the ureters: Grade 1 – limited to the ureter, Grade 2 – reflux up the renal pelvis and calyces, Grade 3 – mild dilatation of the ureter and pelvicalyceal system, Grade 4 – tortuous ureter with moderate dilatation, blunting of fornices but preserved papillary impressions, Grade 5 – severe dilatation of the fornices and pelvicalyceal system, loss of papillary impressions [2]. Each side may have a different grade of reflux.
4. Imaging on completion of voiding: It is used to check for residual urine.

Imaging is especially helpful in neurogenic patients who may show severe bladder trabeculations with diverticula and pseudodiverticula, wide bladder neck and proximal urethra (Figure 7.2) and vesicoureteric reflux. Patients with Parkinson's disease and Multiple sclerosis may show evidence of detrusor-external sphincter dyssynergia [3].

7.5 Advantages of VCU

There are no absolute indications for VCU apart from indications for conventional urodynamics. However, it does provide imaging of the urinary tract which may be desirable

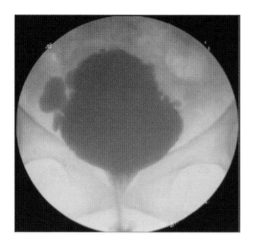

Figure 7.2 Image of the bladder demonstrating diverticula

when undertaken during a functional assessment in complex cases. For complex cases, it provides direct observation of the effect of bladder events on the position and conformation of the bladder neck in relation to the pubic symphysis, bladder neck closure during rest and during rises in intra-abdominal pressure; and direct observation of diverticula of bladder and urethra, vesico-vaginal and urethro-vaginal fistulae, vesicoureteric reflux and voiding events [1]. In the neuropathic bladder, it is valuable for the diagnosis of detrusor external sphincter dyssynergia.

In the 6th International Consultation on Incontinence, it was concluded that VCU may be a reasonable option in the preoperative evaluation of complicated or recurrent urinary incontinence in women [4].

Video recording of the procedures could be used for reviewing complex cases and teaching clinicians to improve their technique and reflect on their practice of urodynamics.

7.6 Limitations of VCU

VCU needs expensive equipment and a dedicated fluoroscopy unit. However, the costs could be justified in complex cases, as it provides useful information in addition to standalone urodynamics.

Suitably trained staff should be available to optimize image quality and reduce the radiation exposure to patients and staff by following appropriate radiological precautions [5].

Anaphylactoid reactions to nonvascular administration of iodinated contrast media are infrequent, but severe reactions can occur unpredictably. VCU should be avoided in patients with known hypersensitivity to iodine-based contrast [6].

Flow rates of the contrast need correction due to the 10% increase on the specific gravity of the iodine in the saline contrast.

VCU is less sensitive in diagnosing detrusor overactivity when compared to ambulatory urodynamics, and, hence, patients with persistent unexplained overactive bladder symptoms should be offered further investigation with ambulatory urodynamics [7].

7.7 Clinical Cases

Case 7.1 Uterovaginal Prolapse

A 54-year-old patient with symptoms of vaginal prolapse, urgency and urgency incontinence requesting surgery for prolapse (Figure 7.3).

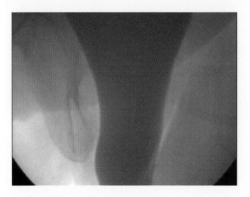

Figure 7.3 Image of a 54-year-old patient with symptoms of vaginal prolapse, urgency and urgency incontinence requesting surgery for prolapse

Case 7.2 Vesicoureteric Reflux

A 66-year-old female presented with voiding dysfunction after a retropubic midurethral tape insertion. Bilateral hydroureters (Figure 7.4) and renal pelvicalyceal dilatation (Figure 7.5) were noted at VCU.

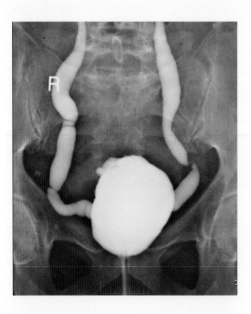

Figure 7.4 Image demonstrating bilateral hydroureters

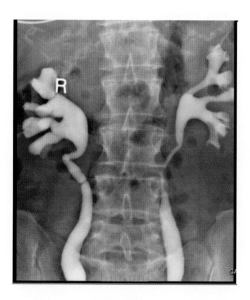

Figure 7.5 Image demonstrating pelvicalyceal dilatation

Case 7.3 Bladder Diverticulum

An 84-year-old female with a vaginal lump, voiding difficultly and stress urinary incontinence. She had a history of total abdominal hysterectomy and a pelvic floor repair. Examination revealed a cystocele and, on VCU, mild stress urinary incontinence and an incidental finding of a bladder diverticulum were noted (Figure 7.6).

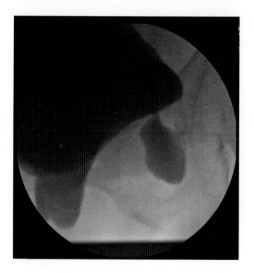

Figure 7.6 Image demonstrating bladder diverticulum

Learning Points

- Set up, catheter insertion and methods to reduce artefacts are similar to conventional urodynamics.

- An iodine-based contrast media such as iohexol is used as a filling medium to allow visualisation of the urinary tract.
- Fluoroscopic images are obtained selectively during filling, at rest, on provocation and during and after voiding.
- Videocystourethrography is indicated in complex cases for direct observation of the effects of bladder events, the position, and conformation of the bladder neck in relation to the pubic symphysis, bladder neck closure during rest and stress, diverticula of the bladder and urethra, vesico-vaginal and urethro-vaginal fistulae, vesicoureteric reflux and voiding events.

References

1. Haylen BT, de Ridder D, Freeman RM, et al. An International Urogynecological Association (IUGA)/International Continence Society (ICS) joint report on the terminology for female pelvic floor dysfunction. *Int Urogynecol J*. 2010;21(1):5–26.

2. Lebowitz RL, Olbing H, Parkkulainen KV, et al. International system of radiographic grading of vesicoureteric reflux. *Pediatr Radiol*. 1985;15(2):105–9.

3. Yamanishi T, Sakakibara R, Uchiyama T. Role of urodynamic studies in the diagnosis and treatment of lower urinary tract symptoms. *Urol Sci*. 2011;22(3):120–8.

4. Abrams P, Cardozo L, Khoury S, Wein AJ, International Continence Society. *6th International Consultation on Incontinence*, Paris; 2017.

5. Giarenis I, Phillips J, Mastoroudes H, et al. Radiation exposure during videourodynamics in women. *Int Urogynecol J*. 2013;24(9):1547–51.

6. Clement O, Webb JAW. Acute adverse reactions to contrast media: mechanisms and prevention. In: Thomsen HS, Webb JAW, eds. *Contrast Media: Safety Issues and ESUR Guidelines*, 3rd ed. Heidelberg, Germany: Springer, 2014:57.

7. Brostorm S, Jennum P, Lose G. Short-term reproducibility of cystometry and pressure/flow micturition studies in healthy women. *Neurourol Urodyn*. 2002;21:457–70.

Chapter 8

Ambulatory Urodynamic Monitoring

Kate Anders and Kal Perkins

8.1 Introduction

Conventional urodynamics (laboratory cystometry) is considered the 'gold standard' for measuring bladder function. However, it is a static short test, typically 20–30 minutes, and is considered 'nonphysiological'. It involves rapid retrograde filling of the bladder in a laboratory setting, which does not always allow reliable reproduction of symptoms. Ambulatory urodynamic monitoring (AUM) relies on physiological bladder filling with natural stressors, including patient mobilisation over a longer time frame, to monitor bladder function which can then be directly compared to presenting symptoms. It is a useful additional test for women in whom conventional urodynamics fails to reproduce or explain the lower urinary tract symptoms of which they complain [1]. AUM is performed through a portable system which allows information to be recorded digitally, and downloaded and reviewed during or at the end of the test. The trace can then be expanded or compressed without loss of information.

8.2 Differences between Ambulatory Urodynamic Monitoring and Conventional Cystometry

AUM is performed in accordance with the International Continence Society (ICS) Standardisation of Ambulatory Urodynamic Monitoring [2]. 'Ambulatory' refers to the nature of the urodynamic monitoring rather than the mobility of the subject and, although it records the same measurements as conventional urodynamics, it differs principally in the following ways:

- AUM is performed over a longer period of time (usually up to 4 hours) and facilitates more than one cycle of bladder filling and voiding.
- It utilises natural bladder filling. (A standard fluid intake, such as 200 ml half-hourly, is recommended.)
- It takes place outside the urodynamics laboratory.
- Its portability allows better reproduction of a patient's normal activities of daily living. These may include manoeuvres tailored specifically to the patient to identify the presence of involuntary detrusor and/or urethral activity and/or to provoke incontinence.

8.3 Indications for Ambulatory Urodynamic Monitoring (AUM)

Indications for AUM are:

- lower urinary tract symptoms which conventional urodynamic investigation fails to reproduce or explain

- neurogenic lower urinary tract dysfunction
- evaluation of therapies for lower urinary tract dysfunction
- assessment of repeated pressure flow studies on voiding (several filling voiding cycles).

8.4 Performing the Test

Care in setting up the equipment, providing advice to patients on the information they should record during the test, and observation of them and troubleshooting are as important in making the diagnosis as the objective measurements obtained, which should not be interpreted in isolation. Checks on signal quality and pressure subtraction are highly important at the start, at regular intervals during the test and again before the test terminates.

8.5 Preparation of the Patient

Information explaining the AUM test including preparation for the test should be sent to patients prior to their appointment. Patients should attend wearing loose comfortable clothing with separate tops and bottoms, and empty their bowel beforehand if possible. Urinalysis is undertaken to exclude urinary tract infection. Concise explanation of the test should be done, and verbal or written consent is taken when the patient attends.

The following would be contraindications:

- acute urinary tract infection
- reduced cognitive ability
- inability to follow instructions
- inability to complete a symptom diary
- severe constipation.

8.6 Equipment and Technique

The following are important components of the equipment required for AUM:

- analysing system and software, urinary flowmeter, electronic incontinence pad or leakage conductance system
- catheter transducers
- patient symptom and event/activity diary.

8.7 The Recording System and Software

The recording unit (Figure 8.1) should be small and lightweight to allow patients freedom of movement. It should have a facility to mark bladder symptoms and events on the trace to support interpretation of the recording which is supplemented with a written or wireless patient diary. Many systems can measure pressures (p_{ves}, p_{abd}, p_{det}, p_{ura}, p_{clos}) with a facility to provide EMG (electromyography). The recorder is connected (either manually or via Bluetooth®) to a urinary flowmeter to allow simultaneous recording of pressure flow. The addition of an electronic pad worn by the patient or a leakage conductance system to supplement patients recording of events and symptoms will facilitate detection of incontinence and diagnosis. Recording units come with an over-the-shoulder strap for patient comfort which should mean minimal interference during physical activities and reduce chances of transducer damage, disconnection or loss.

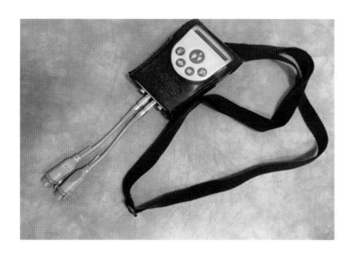

Figure 8.1 Example of recording unit

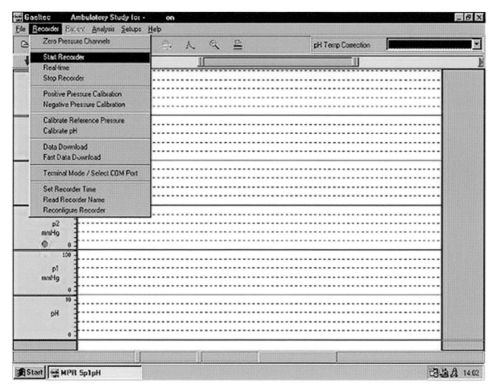

Figure 8.2 Example of software

A high-quality digital memory will allow storage and compression of large amounts of data in addition to allowing for expansion of the recorded trace during the subsequent analysis. Many of the new systems allow more than 24 hours of investigation data to be downloaded, analysed and presented in less than a couple of minutes. Review of recorded data can be made throughout the test using wireless online technology with a Bluetooth® recorder.

An example of software can be seen in Figure 8.2.

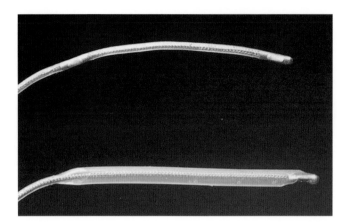

Figure 8.3 Microtip catheter

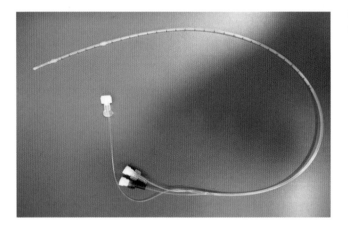

Figure 8.4 Air-charged catheters

8.7.1 The Catheter Transducers

Good quality calibrated catheters to record intravesical and intra-abdominal pressures are vital to ensure robust data for analysis. Solid-state microtip transducer catheters (Figure 8.3) produce fewer movement artefacts compared to water-filled catheters, allowing the patient to have greater mobility which is essential given the ambulatory nature of the test, and have reasonable responsiveness to rapid changes in pressure. The main disadvantages are that they are not of single-use type and therefore require a decontamination process, and they carry a risk of signal loss as there is no fixed reference point. Concerns about decontamination processes and hospital-acquired infection have encouraged the widespread use of single-use transducer catheters in general; commercial manufacturers have sought to improve fluid-filled and air-charged catheter transducers such that many of the AUM systems on the market now use those as viable alternatives to solid-state transducers. Fluid-filled transducers respond quickly to pressure changes but remain sensitive to catheter and patient movement artefacts, however, which can make them less than ideal in an ambulatory setting. Nonetheless, when appropriately secured, they do produce good quality traces. Air-charged catheters (Figure 8.4) are easier to calibrate and have the advantage of

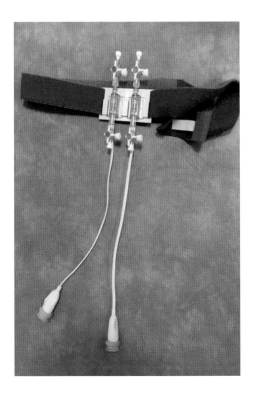

Figure 8.5 External Argon TNR-R pressure transducer and interface cables needed to connect the fluid-filled transducer

being less sensitive to patient and especially catheter movements. However, their response can be slower and relatively damped, especially to rapid pressure changes (e.g. with coughing). Additionally, the catheters are less flexible and are not always well tolerated. This can lead to the test being abandoned early because of symptoms of pain and haematuria which limit their use to 2 hours and decrease the utility of the test. These types of catheters are rarely used in clinical practice.

All catheters must be 'zeroed' before the investigation. Fluid-filled transducers are zeroed to atmospheric pressure at the reference level of the upper border of symphysis pubis and are supported by a belt to keep them in place (Figure 8.5); microtip transducers should be calibrated and zeroed to air before insertion, and air-charged catheters can be zeroed after insertion, but before being 'charged'. Microtip catheters have the pressure-sensitive membrane a few millimetres from the tip. They will record direct contact with any solid material as an apparent change in luminal pressure or artefact; it is possible to mitigate by using a catheter with two transducers (Figure 8.6). As for conventional cystometry, the patient is asked to cough to check for adequate subtraction before the start of the test. Secure transducer fixation of all catheters is essential to minimise artefactual recordings and loss of catheters which is a particular concern because of the movement undertaken by the patient during the test.

8.8 Patient Symptoms and Event Diary

It is vital that the patient understands the nature of the test by providing clear and comprehensive instructions for them to follow because patient compliance is essential for

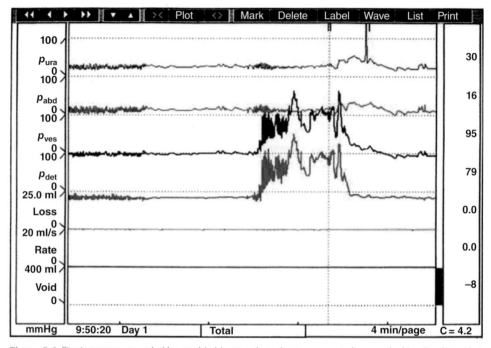

Figure 8.6 Rise in pressure recorded by one bladder transducer (pressure seen in lines marked 'p_{ves}' and 'p_{det}' but not in line marked 'p_{ura}')

a problem-free test and to obtain correct diagnosis. Information and possibly written instructions should be provided on:

- what to do in the event of catheter displacement or hardware failure
- how to complete and use a symptoms and activity diary
- how to use event markers
- how to connect to the flowmeter
- how to manage the electronic urine loss pad.

In conventional cystometry, it is essential that events are annotated and it is even more important in AUM where events do not occur in the same sequence for every patient and are not always witnessed by the urodynamicist. Events are noted in their diary and on the trace by using event markers by the patient and others entered by the urodynamicist. Information noted or recorded during AUM should include the following:

- initiation of voluntary voids
- cessation of voluntary voids
- episodes of urgency
- episodes of discomfort
- provocative manoeuvres
- time and volume of fluid intake
- time and volume of urinary leakage
- time of pad change.

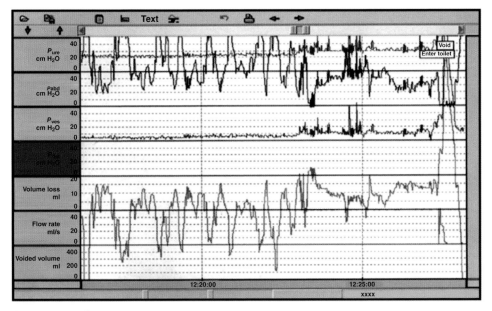

Figure 8.7 Rectal contractions

8.9 Troubleshooting

Constant vigilance, proper calibration, setting up and regular checks of the real-time trace will minimise problems caused by recording measurements while not seeing a constant image. Rectal contraction (Figure 8.7) and general interference can be difficult to avoid and they will not be obvious until the end of the test. Common problems and ways of minimising the risks are listed in Table 8.1.

8.10 Interpretation and Analysis of Results

Newer wireless Bluetooth® techniques make it possible to view data while recording. However, it is important that the urodynamicist performs a real-time check on subtraction at the end of the test to confirm that the pressures have been recorded correctly as part of quality control before removing the catheters. It is important for the patient to be seen for a review of their diary (Figure 8.8) and for event markers or other aspects of the recording to be clarified with the patient at that time. It would be conventional at AUM, for detrusor overactivity only to be diagnosed in association with urgency or with urgency urinary incontinence and if two transducers were placed in the bladder for both to show a rise in pressure (recorded as p_{ura} and p_{ves} on the trace). In conventional cystometry, a diagnosis of detrusor overactivity can be made with pressure rises in the absence of urgency.

8.11 The Clinical Report

A clinical report is produced following discussion of events with the patient, detailed analysis of the traces and review of event markings The clinical report should include the following:

- the duration of recording
- description of signal and data quality

65

Table 8.1 Common problems with AUM and suggestions for minimising the risk of occurrence

Potential problem	Minimising risk
Battery or hardware failure	Use new batteries Regular servicing of hardware
Loss of transducers	Careful fixation of catheters Instruct to patient to inform quickly if there is a loss of catheter
Abdominal interference	Insert transducer above sphincter; e.g. rectal contractions interference is sometimes unavoidable but a clear bowel at start of test will minimise this
Intravesical interference	Careful preparation and insertion of lines
Poor patient compliance	Comprehensive instruction and support
Lack of event marking	Comprehensive instruction
No flow data	Comprehensive instruction on how to use the flowmeter

- fill rate, timing method (and volume of any prior retrograde fill)
- dose and timing of any diuretics
- volume of fluid drunk
- number of voids
- total and range of voided volumes
- episodes of urgency, incontinence and pain
- detrusor activity (frequency, time, duration, amplitude and form)
- pressure and flow analysis
- results of provocative manoeuvres
- reason for early termination.

8.12 Advantages and Disadvantages of AUM

Ambulatory monitoring in clinical practice has become more widely accepted, although controversy remains as to its usefulness in changing management or clinical outcomes.

8.12.1 Advantages

The accommodation of normal activity and physiological rates of bladder filling offers a theoretical advantage when trying to reproduce the patients' normal symptoms and thus increase the likelihood of obtaining a more accurate diagnosis over conventional urodynamics. AUM has an important role in assessment of voiding function with the ability to undertake measurement of repeated pressure flow studies. It also has the advantage over conventional urodynamics in allowing a patient to pass urine in a flowmeter in a private setting when they desire; urinary flow data may be inaccurate or not obtained in the 'inhibited or shy voider' during conventional urodynamics set up in the laboratory.

AMBULATORY URODYNAMICS DIARY

Use the following codes in the diary below and remember to press the
event button when in the toilet. Please use the time displayed on
the front of the recorder.

U = Feeling like you want to/rushing to pass water
P = Passing water

S = Walking up stairs
D = Drinking any other drink, eg. orange, water.

T = Drinking tea or coffee
L = Leaking urine
W = Walking

C = Coughing
R = Sitting

DRINK A CUP OF FLUID AT LEAST EVERY HALF HOUR

Time	Event	Time	Event	Time	Event	Time	Event
09^{10}	Start	11^{13}	W	13^{01}	walk		
09^{12}	Walk			13^{10}	cough leak		
09^{22}	D Sit	11^{20}	C/L				
09^{51}	walk up stairs L	11^{33}	Sit	13^{13}	Pass water		
		11^{37}	Drink Tea	13^{25}	Walking		
09^{59}	P	11^{43}	U	13^{30}	wsency leak		
10^{10}	W	11^{46}	P	13^{34}	Toilet		
10^{23}	R	12^{01}	D				
10^{25}	D	12^{18}	U				
10^{52}	urge P	12^{19}	P				

Pressure lines are checked every hour. This will be done by Sister Anders.
Urogynaecology Unit, King's College Hospital

Figure 8.8 Event diary

8.12.2 Disadvantages

AUM can be labour-intensive and requires longer duration of testing, which limits the number of patients who can be investigated. Patients need to be carefully selected and some patients will not tolerate the catheters for the length of the test. Test analysis is more complicated and it takes extra learning time for someone to become an expert in it; moreover, it requires expensive and additional equipment than that used in conventional cystometry.

8.13 Clinical Cases

Case 8.1 (using water-filled catheters)

Tertiary referral of a 43-year-old woman with symptoms of urgency and urgency incontinence and very occasional leakage on coughing. She had failed conservative treatments. Conventional urodynamics reported as normal (failed to demonstrate any detrusor overactivity or leakage).

At AUM, phasic rise in the vesical and detrusor pressure associated with urgency was noted (recorded as an event marker on both the trace and the patient diary). The trace also shows the patient voiding a few minutes later.

Detrusor overactivity (contractions on p_{det}, p_{ves}) associated with urgency was diagnosed (Figure 8.9).

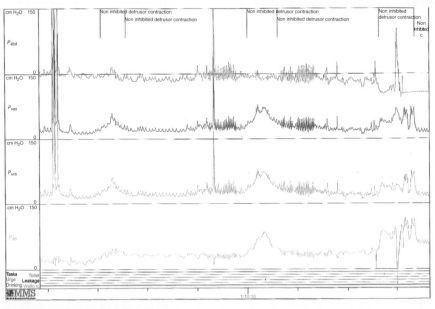

Figure 8.9 Detrusor overactivity (Case 8.1)

Case 8.2 (using air-charged catheters)

A 74-year-old woman with symptoms of urgency and urgency incontinence. Conventional urodynamics failed to reproduce symptoms.

At AUM, phasic rise was noted in vesical and detrusor pressures associated with urgency and leakage. These are marked on the trace with different coloured dots to represent whether the patient is leaking, drinking, walking, has urgency or is passing urine.

Detrusor overactivity (contraction on p_{ura}, p_{det} and p_{ves}) associated with urgency and leaking was diagnosed (Figure 8.10).

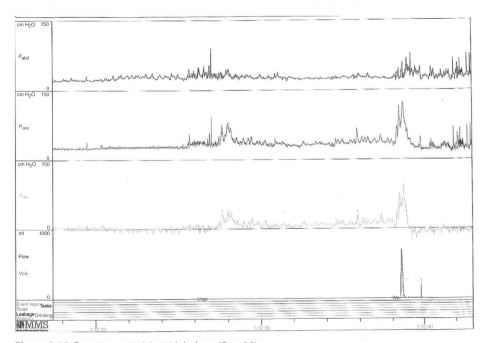

Figure 8.10 Detrusor overactivity with leakage (Case 8.2)

Case 8.3 (Using Microtip Catheters)

A 45-year-old woman who had a transvaginal tape procedure complained of symptoms of stress incontinence when jogging. Conventional urodynamics failed to demonstrate urinary stress incontinence.

The woman was instructed to include a gentle jog in the park while wearing the ambulatory monitoring device. Leakage in the absence of a detrusor contraction was observed with rises in intra-abdominal pressure during jogging marked on the record of events (Figure 8.11).

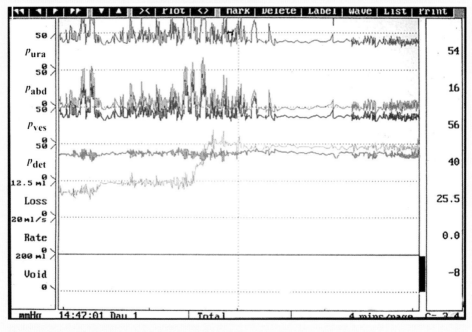

Figure 8.11 Urodynamic stress incontinence (Case 8.3)

Learning Points

- Ambulatory urodynamics is usually undertaken over a 4-hour period, thereby facilitating more than one filling and voiding cycle.
- AUM is undertaken outside the laboratory to mimic the activities of normal daily living.
- Attention to proper calibration and patient ability to follow clear written and verbal instructions are vital in achieving a problem-free test.
- Indications for AUM include failure to reproduce symptoms with conventional tests, neurogenic lower urinary tract dysfunction and repeated flow testing.
- Solid-state microtip transducers are frequently used to measure pressure, but once-only disposable catheters are becoming more common.
- All catheters must be fixed securely to limit artefacts.
- Common problems encountered include poor patient compliance; failure to record events or flow; loss of catheters; and abdominal and vesical interference.

References

1. National Institute of Clinical Excellence (NICE). Urinary Incontinence: the management of urinary incontinence in women: CG171; 2013.

2. van Waalwick van Doorn E, Anders K, Khullar V, et al. Standardisation of ambulatory urodynamic reporting: report of the Standardisation Sub-committee of the International Continence Society for Ambulatory Urodynamic Studies. *Neurourol Urodyn.* 2000;19:113–25.

Urodynamic Artefacts

9

Reeba Oliver and Ranee Thakar

9.1 Introduction

Data quality and documentation of variance are key for urodynamics studies to be valid, and symptoms must be reproduced to be able to make a diagnosis. Accurate reporting requires knowledge of pathophysiological parameters and the ability to detect artefacts. If inaccuracies are discovered, they should be corrected contemporaneously. Spurious and inaccurate observations are known as artefacts. The Oxford dictionary defines artefacts as *something observed in a scientific investigation or experiment that is not naturally present but occurs as a result of the preparative or investigative procedure.'*

These occur because of pitfalls including:

- failure to reproduce symptoms
- observations normally indicating pathology occurring in the absence of disease
- biological variability leading to false negatives
- the wide variation within the physiological range of the normal population.

9.2 Factors Affecting Urodynamic Investigations

Several factors may influence the measurements recorded on the cystometrogram:

- filling medium type, temperature and rate of infusion
- catheter size
- patient position
- testing in an artificial environment
- patient movement and external movement of the catheters
- catheter blockages or expulsion
- communication
- inaccuracies in uroflowmetry
- equipment (all equipment should conform to International Continence Society technical specifications)
- voided volumes less than 150–200 ml.

9.3 Uroflowmetry Artefacts

Artefacts during uroflowmetry may arise owing to several factors, which can be broadly classified into two groups: extracorporeal and intracorporeal.

Extracorporeal causes include:

- flow interference between the collecting funnel and flowmeter
- movement of the stream across the funnel surface

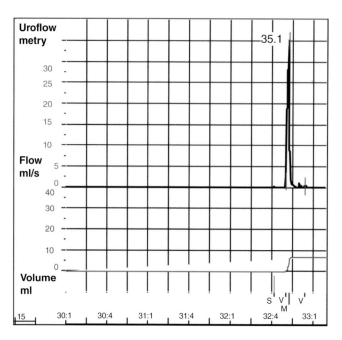

Figure 9.1 Uroflowmetry trace demonstrating changes owing to patient movement. The abrupt spike is recorded by the machine as the maximum flow rate (35.1 ml/s). This is an artefact and gives a falsely high maximum flow rate. The actual maximum flow rate in the region should be read as 20 ml/s.

- momentum artefact due to the momentum of the stream
- patient movement (Figure 9.1).
- very low flow
- time delay

Intracorporeal causes include:

- rapid abdominal straining (Figure 9.2)
- fast and rapid flow (Figure 9.3).
- liquid density error leading to higher flow rates in dehydration.

Although the computerised reading shows a Q_{max} of 35.1 ml/s, manual assessment of flow using smoothed curve denotes the actual Q_{max} of 4 ml/s.

Recommendations to minimise uroflowmetry artefacts include ensuring privacy, checking the report and traces immediately, correcting artefacts manually, and checking that the void was representative of normal.

9.4 Cystometry Artefacts

The setting up of equipment at the beginning of cystometry has been described in Chapters 4 and 6.

Common causes which lead to erroneous observations on the cystometrogram include:

- reference level errors – failure to set zero pressure correctly to atmosphere at the beginning of the test, by placing the transducers at the level of the upper border of the patient's symphysis pubis (Figure 9.4)
- impairment of p_{abd} transmission (Figure 9.5) owing to:

  . faecal loading impairing pressure transmission
  . damping from air in fluid-filled catheters
  . contact of the balloon with the wall of the rectum

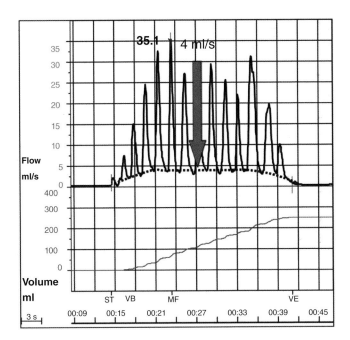

Figure 9.2 Changes in uroflowmetry recording induced by rapid abdominal straining. The solid arrow on the curve drawn denotes the manually read maximum flow rate

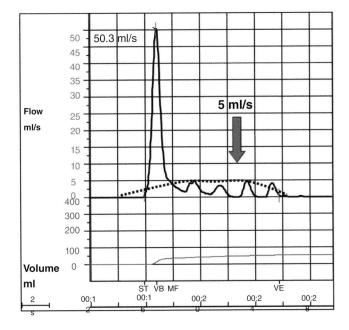

Figure 9.3 Changes in uroflowmetry recording induced by fast and rapid flow; solid arrow on the curve drawn denotes the manually read maximum flow rate. Although the computerised reading shows a Q_{max} 50.3 ml/s, manual assessment of flow using smoothed curve denotes the actual Q_{max} 5 ml/s

- impairment of p_{ves} transmission (Figure 9.6) owing to:
  - catheter not located in the bladder
  - catheter blocked or kinked
  - catheter touching the bladder wall
  - catheter not disconnected from filling line when piggybacked

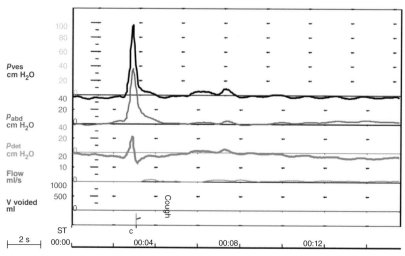

Figure 9.4 Cystometry recording showing incorrect zero pressure caused by setting the catheter-mounted pressure transducers to zero following, rather than prior to, insertion in the body.

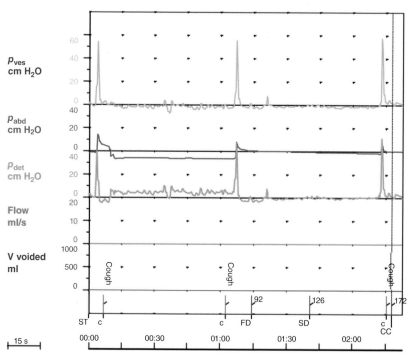

Figure 9.5 Cystometry recording showing impairment of abdominal pressure transmission to the transducer as evidenced by lack of signal response in p_{abd} trace. If abdominal pressure transmission to the transducer is impaired, flush the catheters with water and, if this fails, replace the catheters.

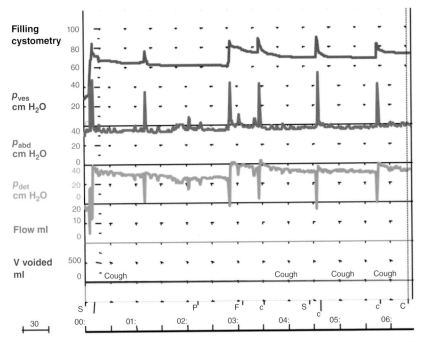

Figure 9.6 Cystometry recording showing impairment of intravesical pressure transmission to the transducer as evidenced by lack of signal response in p_{ves} trace. If intravesical pressure transmission to the transducer is impaired, flush the p_{ves} line (maximum 10 ml) slowly, add fluid to the bladder via filling lumen and check catheter position and reposition if necessary.

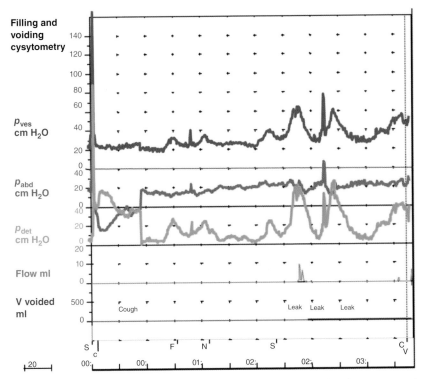

Figure 9.7 Cystometry recording showing a sudden drop in p_{abd}. If a sudden drop or increase in p_{ves} or p_{abd} occurs, ensure that the pressure catheters have not been displaced from the bladder or rectum and reposition them as required.

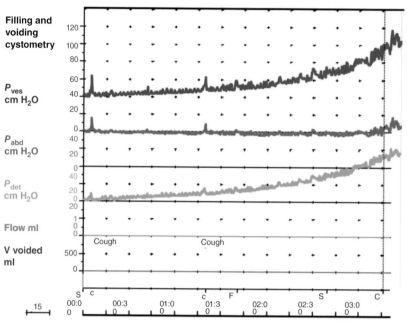

Figure 9.8 Cystometry recording showing a gradual rise in p_{ves} due to fast filling or poor accommodation when approaching cystometric capacity.

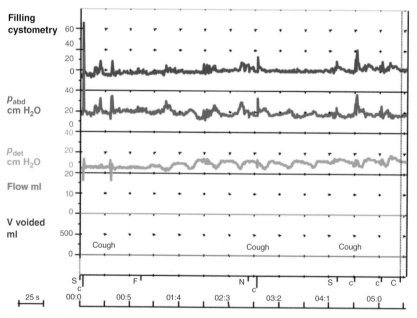

Figure 9.9 Cystometry recording showing rectal contractions. Rectal contractions are seen frequently and defined as multiple fluctuations in abdominal pressure of at least 5 cm H_2O. The clinician must recognise the contractions and not allow them to interfere with the interpretation of the bladder function study.

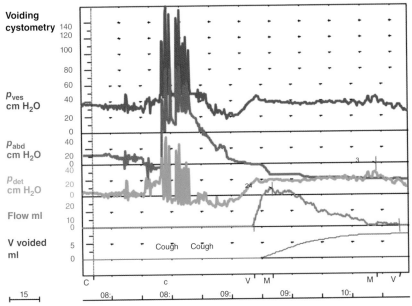

Figure 9.10 Pressure flow recording showing displacement of the rectal pressure transducer. Coughs immediately before and after voiding should be included in the study to ensure that the vesical and rectal pressure transducers are in place

- change in p_{ves} or p_{abd} owing to movement (tube knock) or disconnection of a catheter (Figure 9.7)
- incomplete cough cancellation
- pump vibrations
- line open to syringe
- empty bladder
- empty catheter
- poor cough response
- change in patient position
- gradual rise in p_{ves} owing to fast filling or poor accommodation when approaching cystometric capacity (Figure 9.8)
- physiological artefacts, such as rectal contractions, mirroring in the p_{det} (Figure 9.9)
- baseline drift caused by an air bubble in a fluid-filled line.

9.4.1 Recommendations to Minimise Artefacts

Initial quality checks will prevent the majority of artefacts. Rectify problems with the signal at the beginning of the test and check continuously during the test.

Perform a cough test intermittently during the study. If cough spikes are lost, establish the cause and correct immediately. The p_{abd} and p_{ves} recordings are 'live', showing minor variations of breathing or talking which should not appear in p_{det}.

9.5 Pressure Flow Artefacts

Artefacts may arise during the voiding phase owing to displacement of the vesical or rectal pressure transducer or inadequate pressure transmission (Figure 9.10).

9.5.1 Recommendations to Minimise Pressure Flow Artefacts

Ask patients to cough before and after voiding to confirm correct positioning by checking subtraction on cough spikes.

Learning Points

- Artefacts are spurious and inaccurate urodynamic observations.
- Artefacts arise owing to physical properties of instillant and catheters, patient positioning, artificial environment or technical inaccuracies with recording pressures.
- Artefacts at uroflowmetry are minimised by checking calibration regularly and asking the patient to void normally in private.
- Artefacts during cystometry can be minimised by zeroing transducers to atmospheric pressure, expelling air bubbles, checking subtraction with cough testing before filling, at 1-min intervals during filling and before and after voiding.
- Abdominal and intravesical pressures should show minor 'live' variations during filling which do not appear in the detrusor pressure recording.

Further Reading

Gammie A, D'Ancona C, Kuo HC, Rosier PF. ICS teaching module: artefacts in urodynamic pressure traces (basic module). *Neurourol Urodyn.* 2017;36(1):35–6.

Hogan S, Gammie A, Abrams P. Urodynamic features and artefacts. *Neurourol Urodyn.* 2012;31(7):1104–17.

Rosier PFWM, Schaefer W, Lose G, Goldman HB, Guralnick M. International Continence Society, Good Urodynamic Practices and Terms 2016: urodynamics, uroflowmetry, cystometry, and pressure-flow study. *Neurourol Urodyn.* 2017;36 (5):1243–60.

10

The Assessment of Urethral Function
Supplementary Investigations

Ivilina Pandeva and Mark Slack

10.1 Introduction

The urethra is a complex organ essential for the maintenance of urinary continence. It has always been suggested that as long as the urethral pressure exceeds the one generated by the bladder, continence is maintained. This is a plausible explanation when the patient is at rest but cannot fully explain how this pressure differential is maintained during periods of raised intra-abdominal pressure.

Components of the urethral continence mechanism (Figure 10.1) include the submucosal vasculature, the urethral smooth muscle, the urethral striated sphincter, the bladder neck and the urethral supports. Failure of one or more of these structures can result in incontinence. The striated urethral sphincter extends from 20% to 80% of the urethral length. In the upper two thirds, it has been shown to have a circular orientation and is responsible for a third of the urethral resting pressure. The mucosa and the submucosal vasculature act in tandem to help maintain a tight seal.

Many tests of urethral function have been proposed and the International Continence Society (ICS) has suggested standardisation of the performance of some of these studies and has defined parameters for measurements [1].

It is fair to say that few are used in normal urodynamic practice probably due to inability to guide therapy or provide a predictive value of therapeutic success.

Tests of urethral function include:

- leak point pressure (LPP)
- maximal urethral closure pressure (MUCP)
- fluid bridge test
- Urethral retro-resistance method (URP)

With the exception of the URP, all the other tests require the use of an intra-urethral device to obtain a measurement. It is postulated that this may alter the normal resting anatomy, thus preventing the measurement of the true urethral pressure.

10.2 Urethral Function Tests during Filling Cystometry

Two tests may be included to assess urethral function specifically during filling cystometry:

- vesical or detrusor leak-point pressure estimation
- abdominal leak-point pressure (ALPP)

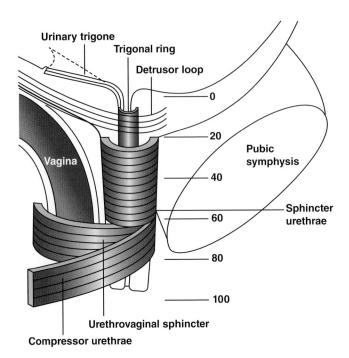

Figure 10.1 Anatomy of the female urethral sphincter (With permission from Taylor & Francis).

10.2.1 Vesical or Detrusor Leak-Point Pressure

Vesical or detrusor leak-point pressure is recorded as the detrusor pressure at the instance of leakage and is considered to be an indirect measure of urethral resistance [2].

10.2.2 Abdominal Leak Point Pressure (ALPP)

ALPP measures the vesical pressure at which leakage occurs during gradual increase in intra-abdominal pressure in the absence of detrusor overactivity. Patients are instructed to produce a graded Valsalva, thereby increasing intra-abdominal pressure while in the upright position at a bladder volume of 200–300 ml and after reduction of pelvic organ prolapse.

10.3 Urethral Function during Voiding Cystometry

Tests of urethral function during voiding cystometry measure the relationship between pressure in the bladder and urine flow rate [1]. Increased detrusor pressure and synchronous, reduced urine flow rates may indicate 'abnormal urethral function'. This may be caused by anatomical abnormalities such as a urethral stricture or urethral overactivity.

10.4 Tests of Urethral Function

Additional tests to assess urethral function specifically may be included when more detailed information on urethral function is desirable.

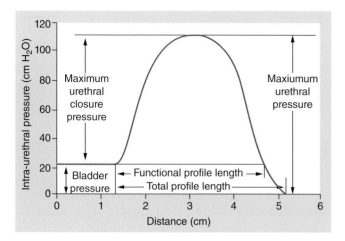

Figure 10.2 Urethral pressure profile parameters (Reproduced with permission from Informa Healthcare).

10.4.1 Urethral Pressure Profilometry (UPP)

UPP provides a graph indicating the intra-luminal pressure along the length of the urethra (Figure 10.2) [2]. A water-perfused catheter, pressure-tip transducer, balloon catheter or air-filled catheter may be used. Profilometry may be performed at rest, during voiding or as a stress test (coughing, straining or Valsalva). The patient positioning is supine (upright position increases maximum urethral closure pressure), at no specified bladder volume and with pelvic organ prolapse reduced. However, it would be standard practice to specify the speed of catheter withdrawal and state reference position for solid-state catheters (usually lateral) and bladder volume during the test. The test is repeated three to six times, for reproducibility. The MUCP measures the passive resistance (or resting tone) of the urethral sphincter.

The parameters recorded are as follows:

- absolute urethral length
- functional urethral length
- maximum urethral pressure
- maximum urethral closure pressure.

When tested in the clinical setting, both MUCP and LPP do not have normal distributions as it is commonly seen with other physiological measures such as height, weight and age. Correlation of the test with symptom severity and treatment outcome is absent.

It is also important to remember that there is poor correlation between MUCP and LPP with neither demonstrating a linear relationship between the two. Patients with severe incontinence as assessed by number of leaks, a visual analogue score (VAS) for bother, a urinary incontinence severity score (UISS) and an incontinence quality of life (I-QOL) were shown to have higher values of MUCP and LPP than patients with less bothersome incontinence [3].

10.4.2 Urethral Retro-Resistance Pressure (URP)

URP has been defined as the pressure required to achieve and maintain an open urethral sphincter [4].

URP is measured by infusing fluid in a retrograde direction against a closed sphincter. The pressure required to open the sphincter is called the urethral retro-resistance pressure (URP). Clinically, this is achieved by placing a cone-shaped metal plug 5 mm into the urethral orifice, creating a seal. The device infuses the fluid into the urethra at a fixed rate of 1 ml/s and displays the pressure required to open and maintain the sphincter in an open position. This technique avoids the use of a urethral catheter and therefore avoids the introduction of a systemic artefact during the test with the hope to produce a more physiological test.

In the studies performed, the large standard deviation in the asymptomatic population meant it had limited application for diagnosis and as a consequence is no longer commercially available [3].

10.4.3 Urethral Pressure Reflectometry (UPR)

UPR is measured using a 5-mm diameter polyurethane bag and a urethral transducer. Urethral pressure and urethral cross-sectional area are simultaneously measured along the entire length of the urethra [3]. Initial studies have compared UPR with UPP and showed a close correlation with maximum urethral closure pressure measurements, with better reproducibility for URP [3].

10.4.4 Ultrasound

Ultrasound is viewed by some as an emerging modality in assessment of pelvic floor dysfunction although its value remains uncertain. It has been used in investigation of stress urinary incontinence for more than 30 years [5]. Technological advances in 3D/4D sonography, coupled with improvements in resolution and quality of images, have contributed to the interest in ultrasonic visualisation of the urethra.

More recently, ultrasound imaging has gained popularity among women and clinicians as a modality to aid diagnosis of complications secondary to mesh implantable materials [6].

The urethra can be visualised by transperineal, introital and transvaginal routes using two-dimensional (2D) or multidimensional ultrasound (3D/4D) [6–9]. Each approach has advantages and disadvantages based on feasibility, image quality, availability of equipment and expertise.

Transperineal ultrasound of the urethra has been described for the evaluation of primary or recurrent stress urinary incontinence following childbirth or previous failed continence surgery by correlating bladder neck position, mobility and hiatal dimension. Although larger hiatal dimension is associated with higher prevalence of stress incontinence, it acts as a surrogate marker and is not diagnostic for the condition [7,8]. Similarly, caudal and posterior bladder neck position and bladder neck mobility are associated with higher rates of stress incontinence; however, none of these findings are able to inform on management options [8].

Assessment of bladder neck mobility by measuring bladder–symphysis distance has been described in the literature. Ultrasound definition for bladder neck descent remains undetermined, but for the diagnosis of hypermobility, a cut-off value of 25 mm has been suggested [9]. The clinical relevance remains to be determined as the previous studies have failed to find a significant difference in bladder neck mobility in women with or without stress urinary incontinence (SUI) [7].

Urethral vascularity has also been assessed by ultrasound with the aim to investigate stress incontinence but again the evidence remains weak and the clinical significance dubious.

There are no studies directly comparing ultrasound to urodynamics or UPP. At present, the level of evidence would indicate that ultrasound evaluation of urethral function should be performed in the context of research setting.

10.5 Indications for Urethral Function Tests

Controversy remains as to the validity and utility of urethral function tests. They are most often used in combination with other urodynamic tests or in a research protocol. There are no absolute indications for these tests in normal clinical practice.

Tests of urethral function may be applied in some clinical circumstances. They may be useful to identify patients with idiopathic voiding dysfunction or idiopathic urinary retention. If urethral instability is suspected, continuous urethral pressure recording, which measures urethral pressure at one point along the urethra for a fixed period of time, is helpful. Tests of urethral function are sometimes used to identify incompetent urethral closure mechanisms, and a pre-operative MUCP of less than 20 cm H_2O may be associated with a higher surgical failure rate.

10.5.1 Potential Advantages of Urethral Function Tests

- An ALPP of less than 60 cm H_2O has been proposed as an indicator of incompetent urethral closure mechanism, although its role in the prediction of outcome is controversial [10].

10.5.2 Limitations of Urethral Function Tests

- Tests of urethral function have low test reproducibility.
- Micro-tip transducers are fragile and expensive and depend upon transducer orientation.
- The introduction of a urethral catheter may prevent the urethra from functioning normally, leading to aberrant readings; for example, urethral pressure is defined as the fluid pressure needed to just open a closed urethra.
- No reference values have been identified to enable differentiation of normal, stress urinary incontinence or detrusor overactivity.
- Successful surgical treatment for stress urinary incontinence does not correlate with changes in UPP parameters.

10.6 Summary

Currently, available methods for assessing urethral pressure have significant limitations and their routine use is not recommended. Most have low test–retest capabilities and fail to discriminate the degree of severity of incontinence. Most importantly, they have no predictive validity and therefore cannot be confidently used in the decision-making process for surgery. In clinical practice, the most commonly used tests are ALPP and MUCP; however, like other urethral function tests, reproducibility is poor which limits their application in clinical setting. At best, urethral function tests can be used as an adjunct to the information gained from conventional cystometry when investigating more complex patients.

Learning Points

- The role of specific tests for urethral function is controversial.
- Urethral pressure profilometry is the most commonly used test of urethral function. It produces a graph of intraluminal pressure along the length of the urethra.
- Poor reproducibility and wide variation of urethral function tests within a normal population limit their application in clinical practice.

References

1. Lose G, Griffiths D, Hosker G, et al. Standardisation of urethral pressure measurement: report from the Standardisation Sub-Committee of the International Continence Society. *Neurourol Urodyn.* 2002;21(3):258–60.

2. Wan J, McGuire EJ, Bloom DA, et al. Stress leak point pressure: a diagnostic tool for incontinent children. *J Urol.* 1993;150(2 Pt 2):700–2.

3. Slack M, Culligan P, Tracey M, et al. Relationship of urethral retro-resistance pressure to urodynamic measurements and incontinence severity. *Neurourol Urodyn.* 2004;23(2):109–14.

4. Slack M, Tracey M, Hunsicker K, et al. Urethral retro-resistance pressure: a new clinical measure of urethral function. *Neurourol Urodyn.* 2004;23(7):656–61.

5. Kohorn EI, Scioscia AL, Jeanty P, et al. Ultrasound cystourethrography by perineal scanning for the assessment of female stress urinary incontinence. *Obstet Gynecol.* 1986;68(2):269–72.

6. Denson L, Shobeiri SA. Three-dimensional endovaginal sonography of synthetic implanted materials in the female pelvic floor. *J Ultrasound Med.* 2014;33(3):521–9.

7. van Veelen A, Schweitzer K, van der Vaart H. Ultrasound assessment of urethral support in women with stress urinary incontinence during and after first pregnancy. *Obstet Gynecol.* 2014;124(2 Pt 1):249–56.

8. Dietz HP. Pelvic floor ultrasound: a review. *Am J Obstet Gynecol.* 2010;202(4):321–34.

9. Dietz HP. Ultrasound imaging of the pelvic floor. Part I: two-dimensional aspects. *Ultrasound Obstet Gynecol.* 2004;23(1):80–92.

10. Lose G, Colstrup H, Saksager K, et al. New probe for measurement of related values of cross-sectional area and pressure in a biological tube. *Med Biol Eng Comput.* 1986;24(5):488–92.

Urodynamics in the Neurological Patient

Laura Thomas and Chris Harding

11.1 Introduction

The term 'neurogenic' bladder is non-specific and applies to any lower urinary tract (LUT) dysfunction which is a consequence of neurological disease. A neurogenic bladder can result in disruption of storage and voiding functions of the LUT depending on the associated neurological pathology, which often (but not always) leads to the LUT symptoms and requires prompt evaluation. Urodynamic testing is frequently undertaken to evaluate such patients, as their disease or injury to the nervous system can have profound consequence. The sequelae of neurological LUT dysfunction can include chronic urinary infection, formation of urinary tract calculi, incontinence, vesico-ureteric reflux, acute kidney injury and chronic kidney disease. There is, therefore, a low threshold for urodynamic investigation within this patient group.

11.2 Patterns of Urodynamic Abnormality

Examples of neurological conditions associated with bladder dysfunction are shown in Table 11.1 [1]. The pattern of LUT dysfunction can often be predicted by the anatomical location of neurological disease or injury. There are three main patterns of LUT dysfunction (Figure 11.1):

- Suprapontine
- Suprasacral (can also be termed Spinal or Infrapontine-Suprasacral)
- Infrasacral

In order to comprehend how the level of lesion impacts on LUT function, it is important to understand the basic processes of filling and voiding. In normality, the bladder stores urine at low pressure with sufficient sphincter activity to maintain continence, and during voiding, the co-ordination of detrusor contraction and sphincter relaxation allows efficient bladder emptying to completion. These functions are complex and require both central and peripheral nervous system involvement. The micturition process can be viewed as specific, important contributions from three distinct central nervous system locations: the higher cerebral cortex which is involved with sensation and decision-making; the brainstem (specifically the pontine micturition centre) which coordinates storage and voiding; and the sacral micturition centre which is involved in detrusor muscle and urinary sphincter contraction/relaxation. Peripheral nervous system contribution is via the parasympathetic, sympathetic and somatic nerves. Parasympathetic nervous system involvement from S2 to S4 spinal cord segments is via pelvic nerves which are responsible for excitatory input to the bladder and lead to detrusor contraction. Sympathetic nervous system input is primarily

Table 11.1 Neurological conditions associated with lower urinary tract dysfunction

Location of Neurological Disease or Injury	Examples
Suprapontine	Cerebrovascular accident (CVA) Multiple sclerosis Head injury Cerebral palsy
Suprasacral	Spinal cord injury Spina bifida Multiple sclerosis
Infrasacral	Cauda equina syndrome Peripheral neuropathy/nerve injury Spina bifida

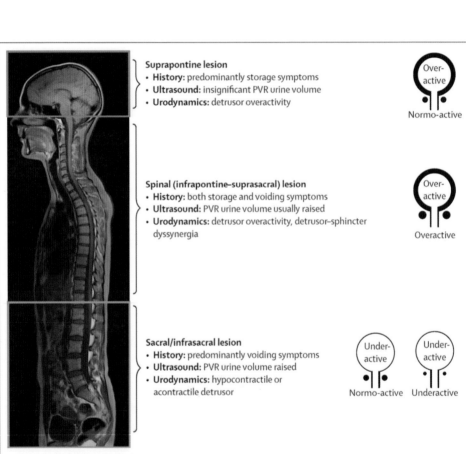

Figure 11.1 Patterns of lower urinary tract dysfunction following neurological disease. (Reproduced from Panicker et al. [2], with permission from Elsevier). Note the common findings from clinical history, ultrasound scanning and urodynamics. The likely pattern of bladder and sphincter activity is also shown (PVR = Post Void Residual).

from T11 to L2 spinal cord segments and causes relaxation of the bladder via the hypogastric nerves. The most important somatic nerves involved in LUT function are the pudendal nerves which supply the striated muscle of the urinary sphincter and also originate from the S2 to S4 spinal cord level.

Supra pontine lesions – disruption to neuronal circuitry above the brain stem.

- Loss of the central inhibition to voiding.
- Reduction in bladder capacity.
- Detrusor overactivity during the filling phase of urodynamic studies.
- If connections between the pontine micturition centre, sacral micturition centre and peripheral nervous system remain intact, then voiding will be normal with unaltered co-ordination of detrusor contraction and sphincter relaxation.
- Sphincter activity is usually normal in these patients.

Suprasacral lesions eliminate both the central inhibition of voiding, as seen in supra-pontine lesions, and local reflex activity below the lesion.

- Detrusor overactivity seen on urodynamic evaluation.
- Possible disturbance to voiding as pontine coordination of detrusor contraction and urethral sphincter relaxation is lost (detrusor–sphincter dyssynergia).
  - very high voiding pressures
  - hydronephrosis and renal dysfunction
  - secondary changes in the bladder becomes hypertrophic and stiffer (urodynamics as loss of compliance)
  - elevated pressures at the end of the filling is an indicator of risk to upper urinary tract.
- Uncoordinated voiding large post-void residual volumes/incomplete bladder emptying.

Infrasacral lesions – trauma to the sacral and subsacral regions.

- Loss of sensation during bladder filling.
- Detrusor acontractility.
- Sometimes, a decrease in bladder compliance which may not be evident in the short to medium term.
- Urethral function dependent on the severity of nerve damage as injury to the pudendal nerve may result in an incompetent urethra which can manifest as urodynamic stress incontinence.

Almost always following a spinal cord injury, there will be a period of acute spinal shock whereby the parasympathetic innervation of the bladder is disrupted rendering the bladder atonic and consequently the patient will experience a period of urinary retention. In these cases, the priority is to ensure patient's upper tracts are safe and this is usually achieved with an indwelling catheter or preferably via the early establishment of intermittent catheterisation. Urodynamics are normally delayed until the period of spinal shock has subsided (6–12 weeks).

11.3 Urodynamic Technique

The role of urodynamics in neurological patients is to identify any underlying detrusor or sphincter abnormalities, in order to formulate appropriate treatment plans and reduce possible risk to upper urinary tracts. Urological assessment of the LUTs is fundamentally similar for neurological and non-neurological patients. It is still important to take an in-depth history, inclusive of bladder diaries and validated symptom questionnaires, and perform a thorough examination which should include a neurological assessment. Careful prior consideration needs to be given to the possible urodynamic findings and the manner in which the test has to be conducted, which actually needs to be tailored to the individual patient within their physical and mental capabilities.

Before any invasive urodynamic procedure is conducted, urinalysis should be performed and hospital guidelines on appropriate antibiotic administration should be followed. Patients with neurogenic LUT dysfunction can often be at high risk for developing severe urinary tract infections.

11.3.1 Free Flow (Uroflowmetry)

- Free flo (uroflowmetry) may not be possible with all patients, and some patients may only be able to void in a particular position and equipment should be arranged accordingly.
- Current opinion would not recommend draining any residual volume before beginning filling cystometry and as such an ultrasound scan may be useful in determining bladder residual volume.
- An exception to the above conditions is patients who are already performing clean intermittent catheterisation who would usually have their bladder emptied after voiding.

11.3.2 Filling Cystometry

- Speed of infusion should be slow and constantly monitored.
- Filling too fast has the potential to provoke detrusor overactivity or create artificial changes in the bladder compliance.
- In those circumstances, those findings may mask the patient's true physiology and yield erroneous results from the urodynamic study.
- Infusion of fluid during the filling phase can be stopped and any changes in resting pressures should be monitored.
- A drop in vesical pressure when filling is suspended may indicate that apparent changes in compliance are likely due to the filling rate exceeding the bladder's visco-elastic capability rather than true loss of compliance. In this scenario, filling should be re-commenced at a slower rate.

11.3.3 Voiding Cystometry (Pressure Flow Study)

- The patient should be allowed to void in a position that is normal and comfortable for them. Departments who perform large numbers of complex urodynamics may benefit from couches that can be manipulated to create a position conducive to the patient's normal voiding position.
- In those patients who are unable to sit to void, a mechanism which is similar to that of a drain pipe can be used, which allows the urine to reach a flow meter albeit with a delay.

11.3.4 Considerations

Patients with spinal injuries at T6 or above are at risk of autonomic dysreflexia (AD), a potentially life-threating condition caused by an uncontrolled autonomic response most commonly as a result of a peripheral stimulus such as bladder or bowel distention.

- Signs of AD include hypertension, pounding headache, changes in skin colour – either flushing or blotching – above the height of the injury.
- The danger in this situation is the uncontrolled hypertension, and between 36.7 and 77.8% of patients with T6 or higher lesions experience an episode of AD during urodynamic assessment [3].
- Regularly monitor blood pressure throughout urodynamics in neurological patients.
- Have access to Nifedipine or GTN spray, as those patients who experience an episode of AD may require these medications.
- Guidelines recommend the use of fluoroscopy (video urodynamics) to provide information regarding the presence of vesico-ureteric reflux.
- Additional procedures include urethral pressure profilometry (UPP), abdominal leak point pressures (ALPP) or electromyography (EMG).
- Long-term monitoring of urinary symptoms can be through ambulatory urodynamics if it was not possible to reproduce their symptoms during initial video urodynamics.

All good urodynamic tests are performed interactively with the patient and should be tailored to create an environment of filling and voiding which is as normal to the patient's usual situation as possible. Additional to patients' physical capabilities, it is also imperative that patient's cognitive ability, namely comprehension and understanding, is considered. All parts of the procedure should be explained in full and therefore sufficient time needs to be given to these appointments to allow for a worthwhile test. Any concerns regarding the integrity of the urodynamic results should be addressed during the test, not retrospectively.

11.4 Reporting

The following measurements or observations represent the minimum information which should be recorded when urodynamics are undertaken in the neurological patient:

- Sensation
  - Record the bladder volumes at the first desire to void and strong desire to void, and document the cystometric capacity.
  - Is sensation increased, reduced or absent?

- Storage
  - Document the bladder volumes at the start and end of the filling phase and record the corresponding detrusor pressures.
  - Is there evidence of phasic detrusor activity seen during filling? (neurogenic detrusor overactivity).
  - Is there evidence of loss of bladder compliance?

- Incontinence
  - Record any episodes of incontinence and annotate urodynamic traces.

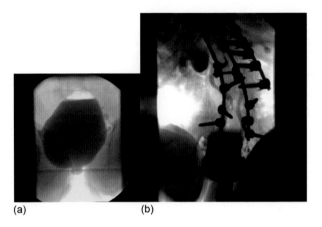

Figure 11.2 (a) Video fluoroscopy from a urodynamic study of a female patient with detrusor–sphincter dyssynergia; note the multiple bladder diverticula and the characteristic dilatation of the proximal urethra. (b) Video fluoroscopy from a urodynamic study of a male patient with detrusor–sphincter dyssynergia; note the multiple bladder diverticula, the characteristic dilatation of the proximal urethra, bilateral vesico-ureteric reflux and the metalwork from previous spinal surgery.

(a)   (b)

- Leak point pressures
    - Abdominal (valsalva) leak point pressure: intravesical pressure at which urine leakage is observed [4].
    - Values of <60 cm H_2O^{-1} are indicative of intrinsic sphincter deficiency.
    - The detrusor leak point pressure: the lowest detrusor pressure at which urine leakage occurs in the absence of a detrusor contraction or increased abdominal pressure [4]. Estimate the likelihood of upper urinary tract complications as a result of loss of compliance. A figure of >40 cm H_2O^{-1} indicator of likely upper tract complications [5].

- Voiding
    - Document the detrusor pressure at maximum flow and the corresponding maximum urine flow rate.
    - Are the detrusor contractions well-sustained or fluctuant?
    - Was voiding voluntary or involuntary?
    - Document the presence of abdominal straining.
    - Record any incomplete bladder emptying, including an estimation of the post-void volume.
    - Document any evidence of detrusor–sphincter dyssynergia.

- Radiological abnormalities (see Figure 11.2)
    - The structure of the bladder outlet. Evidence of mechanical obstruction? Proximal urethra dilated? Does the outlet change during voiding (suggestive of detrusor–sphincter dyssynergia)?
    - The conformation of the bladder, including a 'control' image, evidence of bladder calculi, bladder trabeculation or diverticula?
    - Is there any evidence of vesico-ureteric reflux and if so what grade is it and is it bilateral or unilateral?

A report summary should detail
- Abnormalities of storage
- Abnormalities of voiding
- Radiographic (structural) abnormalities.

Learning Points

- Urodynamics in neurological patients is important and highly specialised.
- Management decisions are often directly linked to Urodynamic assessment findings and therefore accuracy and detail of the test cannot be overstated.

References

1. National Institute for Health and Care Excellence (NICE). Clinical Guideline 148. Urinary incontinence in neurological disease: assessment and management; 2012. www.nice.org.uk/guidance/cg148

2. Panicker JN, Fowler CJ, Kessler TM. Lower urinary tract dysfunction in the neurological patient: clinical assessment and management. *Lancet Neurol.* 2015;14 (7):720–32.

3. Liu N, Zhou M, Biering-Sørensen F, Krassioukov AV. Iatrogenic urological triggers of autonomic dysreflexia: a systematic review. *Spinal Cord.* 2015;53:500–9.

4. Abrams P, Cardozo L, Fall M, et al. The standardisation of terminology of lower urinary tract function: Report from the Standardisation Sub-committee of the International Continence Society. *Neurourol Urodyn.* 2002;21:167–78.

5. McGuire EJ, Woodside JR, Borden TA, et al. Prognostic value of urodynamic testing in myelodysplastic patients. *J Urol.* 1981;126:205–9.

Urodynamic Terminology
United Kingdom Continence Society: Minimal Standards for Urodynamics, 2018

Paul Abrams

12.1 Introduction

The publication 'United Kingdom Continence Society: Minimum Standards for Urodynamic Studies, 2018' was commissioned by the UK Continence Society (UKCS), to replace the Joint statement on minimum standards for urodynamic practice in the United Kingdom: Report of the urodynamic training and accreditation steering group (published in April 2009 by the UKCS). The 2009 document has been completely rewritten with the prime aim of providing information, advice and guidance to help with best practice in urodynamic study services. The full version of the 2018 document has been accepted and published in *Neurourology and Urodynamics* [1].This work is a shortened version of the document and appears with the permission of NAU under a joint copyright agreement between NAU and UKCS.

Urodynamics have developed in the United Kingdom since the early 1970s, thanks to the scientific efforts of a range of healthcare professionals (HCPs). These include urologists, gynaecologists, clinical scientists, nurses and technicians. As of this writing (2018), UDS are still performed by a range of HCPs, some of whom have received no formal UDS training, largely because they started urodynamic practice before there was any formal urodynamic training. However, today it is expected that all those starting to perform UDS should have received formal training and assessment.

There are uncomfortable deficiencies in the regulation of UD services that undoubtedly harm patients. Indeed, there are currently no statutory requirements for the performance of urodynamic testing and little or no quality assurance, when compared to the essential regulations for treatment modalities from medicinal products to surgical procedures. The UKCS believes that it is unacceptable that UDS, an invasive test and an important part of the patient pathway for many men, women and children, will, if inexpertly performed, lead to some patients being denied necessary treatment, and others being subjected to treatments they cannot, or are unlikely to, benefit from. The UKCS is the major multidisciplinary group of HCPs, in the United Kingdom, dedicated to helping those suffering from lower urinary tract dysfunction (LUTD) such as urinary incontinence, and is determined to improve the care of patients.

It is intended for use by the doctors, nurses and scientists who provide urodynamic services, and as information to those who commission urodynamic services for their patients across the United Kingdom. The document may also help urodynamic services in other countries. However, readers are advised that practices may vary outside the United Kingdom.

The information in this booklet has been compiled from professional sources. While every effort has been made to ensure that the publication provides accurate and expert information and guidance, it is impossible to predict all the circumstances in which it may be used.

The document was developed through a consensus approach predominantly via membership of the UKCS Working Group: clinical scientists, nurses, adult and paediatric urologists, and urogynaecologists, each of who has extensive personal practical experience of performing UDS.

The UKCS is pleased that the following UK organisations have reviewed and endorsed the document: Association for Continence Advice; British Association of Paediatric Urologists; British Association of Urological Nurses; British Association of Urological Surgeons (BAUS); BAUS Section of Female, Neuro Urology, and Urodynamics; British Society of Urogynaecologists; Institute of Physics and Engineering in Medicine; Royal College of Nursing, Continence Forum; Royal College of Obstetricians and Gynaecologists; and the Urogynaecology Nurse Specialist Committee. The document has also been reviewed and endorsed by the International Continence Society.

The aim of the document is to improve the care of patients with LUTD by helping to ensure that the urodynamic studies (UDS) used in their assessment are of the highest possible quality, by providing clear minimum standards for UDS, to the urologists, gynaecologists, clinical scientists, nurses and technicians responsible for carrying out UDS.

The document has the following sections:

- Principal indications for UDS in children, women, men and neurological patients
- Minimum standards for a urodynamic unit
- Urodynamic skill sets
- The urodynamic patient pathway
- Urodynamic techniques
- Guidance for commissioners and providers of urodynamic services
- General recommendations

The full report has appendices which can be found on the UKCS website: Urodynamics antibiotics policy; Urodynamics patient leaflets for children, women, men, neurological patients, and patients after urodynamics; Bladder diary and symptom questionnaires (ICIQ-BD – International Consultation on Incontinence Questionnaire Bladder Diary; ICIQ-FLUTS – International Consultation on Incontinence Questionnaire Female Lower Urinary Tract Symptom; ICIQ-MLUTS – International Consultation on Incontinence Questionnaire Male Lower Urinary Tract Symptoms); a template urodynamics report; Skills for health competencies; and Training and CPD details for urodynamics staff.

12.2 Principal Indications for UDS in Children, Women, Men and Neurological Patients

This section does not seek to provide an exhaustive list that includes every possible indication, but to list those indications that include perhaps 90% of those having UDS.

In general, urodynamics are only used if:

- Lifestyle changes and drug therapy have not provided adequate improvement in the individual's quality of life, and further therapy such as surgery is being contemplated after discussion with the patient, and/or carer.

- There are factors that might lead to deterioration in lower urinary tract (LUT) function with possible consequences for the upper urinary tract, particularly in children and some patients with neurogenic LUT dysfunction.

Therefore, it follows that UDS are not indicated when:

- the patient has not been treated using lifestyle changes and drug therapy, when appropriate;
- the patient does not wish to consider surgical management after failed conservative treatment;
- UDS is not likely to provide information that will change the management of that patient.

In *children*, the most frequent indications for UDS are as follows: congenital neurological conditions, including spina bifida and sacral agenesis; congenital structural conditions, including posterior urethral valves, anorectal malformations and bladder exstrophy; dysfunctional voiding; and failed overactive bladder (OAB) treatment prior to Botulinum toxin type A (BTXA) or sacral nerve stimulation.

In *women*: prior to surgery for bothersome stress incontinence; women with pelvic organ prolapse (POP) and urinary symptoms considering surgery and women with new onset lower urinary tract symptoms (LUTS) post pelvic floor surgery; idiopathic voiding dysfunction/urinary retention; and failed OAB treatment prior to BTXA or sacral nerve stimulation.

In *men*: prior to possible surgery for suspected prostatic obstruction; post-prostatectomy stress incontinence; in younger men (e.g. <45 years) with voiding symptoms/history of retention; and failed OAB treatment prior to BTXA or sacral nerve stimulation.

In *neurological patients*, congenital or acquired neurological conditions with a risk of upper tract deterioration (e.g. spinal cord injured patient and spina bifida); and significant LUTS, including incontinence, that have not responded to conservative management.

12.3 Minimum Standards for a Urodynamic Unit

The key features of a urodynamic unit (UDU) include:

- *Director of the UDU*: A director should be appointed who is usually a consultant urologist specialising in functional urology or a consultant urogynaecologist. However, the Director may be a consultant nurse or clinical scientist. The director has many roles primarily aimed at ensuring that the patient has appropriate and safe high-quality UDS.

These roles include: determining the scope of the UDU defined by whether the UDU has a secondary, tertiary or specialist referral pattern; integrating the UDU into the hospital environment; ensuring that the UD staff have the necessary education, training and CPD, to have the necessary skill sets exist to ensure high-quality UDS; to ensure that urodynamic equipment is fit for purpose and maintained; and to lead regular appropriate multi-disciplinary team and audit meetings.

- *UDU referral patterns:* Secondary care units offer a local service with basic UDS for men and/or women without complex problems; tertiary care unit offer a service that also includes video UDS (VUDS), urethral function studies and ambulatory UDS for men and/or women with complex problems, from a wider geographical area; and specialist regional units offer the full range of UD tests to a well-defined population, such as children or spinal cord injury patients.

- *Integration in the hospital environment:* this includes collaboration with the organisation's Radiology, Information Technology (IT) and Medical Physics departments.
- *UDU clinical environment:* certain features are essential; there must be adequate space for equipment/consumable storage, and consultation, as well as accessibility for wheelchairs/hoists, etc.; patient privacy and dignity is important with proper changing and toilet facilities; a disposal facility for body fluids; and a proper couch for examination.
- *Administrative support* is needed for an effective UDU, including: requirements for service provision, including processing of clinical notes and dictation on patients and establishment and maintenance of a UD database; and making appointments and ensuring that all disposable equipment is available and patient information leaflets in stock.

UDU staffing: UDS are delivered in a variety of models, but all have the same common principles.

- Patient safety and well-being necessitate there being two HCPs at each UDS. In general, this allows one to concentrate on the technical aspects of the test whilst the second person talks with the patient and interprets symptoms with urodynamic findings, during the test. In addition, if there is an unexpected event, such as a syncopal attack (fainting), then the patient can be properly cared for. All staff need to be aware of local policies including infection control, manual handling, intimate examination and chaperoning.
- The technical aspects of UDS can be provided by a nurse, technologist or a suitably trained doctor.
- The clinical aspects of UDS can also be provided by a nurse, clinical scientist or a suitably trained doctor.
- During VUDS, it may also be necessary to have radiology staff present.

12.3.1 Training and CPD for UD Staff

- The UKCS takes the view that those who have been formally trained best serve patients. Training should be based on indicative minimum numbers of UDS performed, combined with structured competence assessments which document the trainees' progress until they have acquired the competence needed to work independently. Assessment of competence varies with specialty but may include a log of cases, objective structured assessments of training, direct observations of procedure, mini clinical examination and case-based discussions, including analyses of traces.
- Practice levels for consultant staff, or equivalent, working in UDUs is seen as an essential part of CPD and regular sessions in the UDU are essential, and a minimum of 12 sessions per year, once staff are fully trained, is essential to maintaining standards.
- *Urodynamic papers and books:* There are a number of important papers that should be read by all those undertaking UDS, and responsible for either the technical, clinical, or both aspects of UDS. In addition, HCPs intending to perform UDS should read one of the published books on UDS. These papers and books provide the principal information sources for all UDS.

- ICS Terminology 2002 [2].
- Urodynamic features and artefacts 2012 [3].
- ICS Equipment Performance 2014 [4].
- International Continence Society: Good Urodynamic Practices and Terms 2016 [5].
- *Urodynamics Made Easy* [6].
- *Urodynamics* [7].
- International Children's Continence Society Standardization Report on Urodynamic Studies of the Lower Urinary Tract in Children [8].
- The standardization of terminology of lower urinary tract function in children and adolescents: Update report from the standardization committee of the International Children's Continence Society [9].
- *Clinical Urodynamics in Childhood and Adolescence* [10].

  - *Urodynamic Courses:* Urodynamic courses are very valuable and should be chosen by the HCPs according to their experience and the types of patients they deal with or will be investigating. These courses should be led by doctors, nurses and clinical scientists with both practical and academic knowledge of UDS: they should not be industry led. Industry has a very valuable part to play in urodynamic courses by providing equipment for the attendees to see and handle. The organisers should endeavour to make available UD equipment from more than one company.

12.4 Urodynamic Skill Sets

12.4.1 Essential Technical Skills

Essential technical skills refer to the skills needed to run the technical aspects of a UDS. This skill set is used to deliver technical excellence in UDS by a technologist, nurse, clinical scientist or doctor who has been fully trained. The skill set includes:

- A relationship with the Medical Physics or Clinical Engineering department/ manufacturers with both an annual planned preventative maintenance arrangement, and ability to arrange ad hoc visits, if necessary, in the event of equipment problems.
- Maintain the urodynamic equipment (pressure transducers, flow meters, weight transducers and infusion devices) on a day-to-day basis.
- Be able to carry out daily/weekly calibration checks of the UD equipment.
- Have a sound knowledge of the physiological range for all the main UD measurements: urine flow, and abdominal, urethral, and vesical pressures, as this information is the basis from which high-quality traces result.
- Produce a high-quality trace from the technical point of view, with proper quality control according to ICS 2016 (see Section 12.4.2).
- Recognise and correct artefacts that occur during UDS, some of which will be physiological, and others mechanical/electrical coming from the equipment, described in a comprehensive paper by Hogan et al. [3].
- Be able to annotate traces correctly, so that others who were not present at the UDS can properly understand the recordings.

12.4.2 Essential Clinical Skills

A range of skills and ability is necessary to deliver the clinical aspects of a UDS and to perform an excellent clinical study to each patient. They may be possessed by a nurse, clinical scientist or doctor who has been trained *according to UKCS 2018 standards*. They include:

- Sound knowledge of the anatomy and physiology of the lower urinary tract, and the principle conditions affecting the bladder and urethra (LUTD).
- Clinical assessment of patients on the day of the UDS, and, in particular, confirmation of the urodynamic questions to be answered.
- Insertion of the urodynamic catheters using the aseptic non-touch technique (bladder) and a clean technique (bowel or vagina).
- During insertion of the rectal catheter, ensuring, by digital examination, that the patient does not have a loaded rectum as this is likely to influence the UD findings.
- Having a continuous dialogue with the patient in order to assess whether their symptoms are reproduced during the UDS.
- Assuring quality control during the UDS.
- Altering technique, if need be, during the investigation.
- Dealing with patient problems such as fainting: this is an example of a situation that demands that two HCPs are present during all UDS.
- Interpreting the UD tracing and reaching one or more urodynamic diagnoses, in light of the urodynamic questions asked.
- Stating whether or not the patient's symptoms have been reproduced during UDS.
- Having an outline discussion with the patient at the end of UDS, covering both the diagnosis and a description of possible treatment options (setting a management plan in the light of the question(s) asked).
- If the HCP at UDS is the clinician responsible for delivering the treatment, the discussion will be in detail. If not, the detailed discussion will occur at a later date with the responsible consultant who would be expected to be trained in urodynamics, and a member of the local urodynamic MDT.
- NOTE: the UKCS considers that the UD diagnosis should be made at the time of the UDS and does not think it is appropriate for the diagnosis to be made at a remote location, by a clinician without access to the patient, perhaps delayed by a considerable period of time.
- Being part of, and attending the MDT
  - Urodynamic equipment
    - *Recommended equipment:* Urodynamics is very dependent upon the appropriate use of good quality equipment. Table 12.1 lists the equipment recommended for different levels of urodynamic service. A guide to the specifications for this equipment can be found in the ICS guidelines for urodynamic equipment performance.
      - *Maintenance routines and regular checks:* maintenance of urodynamic equipment and checks of its proper calibration are essential, not just for

Table 12.1 Recommended equipment for different urodynamic investigations

Type of Service	Equipment Required
Urine flow recording	Uroflowmeter Commode (female)/stand (male) Ultrasound machine for measurement of post-void residual volume
Standard UDS: Filling cystometry and pressure-flow study of voiding	Uroflowmeter Commode (female)/stand (male) Pressure transducer mounting stand Urodynamic equipment with two pressure transducers and infusion pump, and, if required, electromyography (EMG) recording channel
VUDS (additional requirements to above)	Imaging apparatus (image intensifier, fixed X-ray unit or ultrasound machine) Urodynamic equipment with video capture included
Urethral function studies	Motorised withdrawal unit and pump for urethral pressure profilometry Three pressure channels required if urethral pressure is also measured while filling/voiding
Ambulatory UDS	Ambulatory urodynamic equipment (two pressure channels, data logger, linked flowmeter, computer for data download and analysis)

patient safety but also for a reliable urodynamic measurement. Responsibility for this is equally that of the UD HCPs, as well as the technical support. These checks should be planned and recorded and include:

○ regular checks of calibration of the flowmeter (checking the accuracy of a known volume)

○ regular checks of calibration of pressure transducers (checking, e.g., that 0–50 cm H_2O is registered correctly)

○ computer software and hardware updates and maintenance

○ electrical safety tests, normally every year or two

○ additional technical support from medical physics or clinical engineering department, or from manufacturer, under contract if necessary

– Detailed technical and operational considerations are outlined in the *'Buyers' Guide for Urodynamic Equipment'*, published by the Department of Health (www.nhscep.useconnect.co.uk)

. *Regular audit* allows the periodic confirmation of quality in UDUs. The following audits are recommended: the appropriateness of UD referrals; post-UDS urinary traction infection (UTIs); quality control of UD traces (see Table 12.2); outcome of UDS in terms of whether the patient's symptoms were reproduced, and the defined urodynamic questions answered; effect of UDS on clinical outcome; and patient experience/satisfaction.

Table 12.2 Checklist for assessing quality in UD recordings

Display	Are intravesical pressure (p_{ves}), abdominal pressure (p_{abd}) and detrusor pressure (p_{det}) and flow traces all present, scaled and labelled?
	Are infused and voided volume figures or graph displayed?
	Do the printing scales permit clear display of all trace features?
Quality Control	Are p_{ves} and p_{abd} zeroed to atmosphere (both >0 cm H_2O after zeroing and connection to patient)?
	Are resting p_{ves} and p_{abd} in the range 5–20 cm H_2O (supine), 15–40 cm H_2O (seated) and 30–50 cm H_2O (standing)?
	Is the resting p_{det} between −5 and +5 cm H_2O?
	Are live signals visible throughout the test (or after any correction) on p_{abd} and p_{ves}, but not visible on p_{det}?
	Are cough tests done: before filling, regularly during filling, before and after voiding?
	Are the smaller cough test peaks ≥70% of the larger peaks in both p_{ves} and p_{abd} traces, or corrected if not?
	Is poor compliance seen, and if so, was the pump stopped until pressure stabilised?
	Is there abnormal steady pressure descent and was it corrected?
Flows (both pressure-flows and free flows)	Is the point of maximum flow (Q_{max}) marked or reported on all traces where flow occurs?
	Is the Q_{max} marker moved away from artefacts?
	Are voided volume, post-void residual, flow time and voiding time recorded being corrected for any involuntary leakage during filling?
Markers	Are any involuntary detrusor contractions (DO), leaks, position changes, VLPP or stress tests marked as such?
	Is 'permission to void' marked?
	Are all values at markers clear, either from the trace or the table of events?
	Are all values used in diagnosis free from artefact?

12.5 The Urodynamic Patient Pathway

There are a number of important aspects that help to ensure that patients have a satisfactory experience:

- *Patient referral:* each referral must include:
  - The 'Urodynamic Questions' that the referring clinician wants answered, for example, 'this man has a reduced urine flow rate and has persistent bothersome LUTS and wishes to be considered for trans-urethral resection of prostate (TURP); can you confirm the presence of obstruction?'

- Current medication for LUTD with drug dosage and length of treatment. Opinions vary as to whether patients should stop LUTD drugs before UDS, and there is no clear evidence to guide this decision. This emphasises the importance of knowing which drugs patients are taking at the time of UDS.
- Relevant physical findings: in women, the results of a vaginal examination to exclude pelvic abnormalities should be noted, including details of any pelvic organ prolapse and oestrogenisation of the vagina. However, the urodynamic HCP may be a clinical scientist who would not be expected to do a pelvic examination where appropriate: this issue needs to be resolved locally.
- Results of screening urine flow studies (UFS), with post-void residual (PVR) measurement, which should be done prior to UDS in all men, and in women with voiding symptoms. Furthermore, the data from UFS are important for comparison with the flow measurements during the UD pressure-flow study (PFS).
- A statement as to whether the patient is one at high risk of getting a urinary tract infection (UTI) from the UDS. If so, then the local urodynamic antibiotic policy should be followed.

- *Patient preparation includes: sending information about UDS to the patients; asking the patients to complete a symptom questionnaire* (the ICIQ-FLUTS for women and the ICIQ-MLUTS for men are recommended) *and complete a 3-day bladder diary (ICIQ-BD); and give antibiotic prophylaxis if indicated.*
  - *Day of the urodynamic study*
  - *Safeguarding the patient, including:* ensuring that any necessary antibiotic prophylaxis has been taken appropriately; providing an appropriate chaperone, and for a child, ensuring that the local policy for safeguarding children is followed; providing a clinical environment that maintains the maximum possible privacy and dignity, with screens for changing, and availability of single-sex changing areas/ toilets in line with local policy.
  - *Initial testing and physical examination*

    - Ask the patient to empty his or her bladder and do a flow study, recording maximum urine flow rate (Q_{max}), volume voided (VV) and post-void residual urine volume (PVR).
    - Perform the dipstick test on voided urine to exclude infection, and if positive, follow the local urodynamic antibiotics policy.
    - Examine the patient: *Abdominal*, to exclude a palpable bladder after voiding and obvious masses; *Perineal* inspection for sensation, skin condition and visible pelvic floor contraction; *Rectal* examination to assess anal tone, pelvic floor contraction and to exclude faecal loading; Staff who are trained to do so: for women not previously examined, perform. ... *In women*, perform vaginal examination for pelvic abnormalities and record details of any pelvic organ prolapse (POP) and oestrogenisation of the vagina; Simple *neurological* testing of lower limbs to assess sensation, muscle strength and reflexes may be indicated.

  - Urodynamic Studies

    - UDS vary in their complexity and their frequency of use. 'Standard UDS' include filling cystometry and a pressure-flow study of voiding, and are applicable for the large majority of men and women coming to a UDU. The largest patient group in whom UDS is indicated is women with urinary symptoms. Men with urinary symptoms comprise the second largest group of patients referred for UDS, with significantly smaller numbers of patients with neurological disease and children undergoing this test. Video and ambulatory UDS are indicated in much smaller sub-groups of patients.

– As a general rule, UDS are indicated in patients when lifestyle interventions and drug therapy have failed to alleviate bothersome symptoms, and invasive surgical treatment is being considered. In an important minority of patients, UDS are indicated if there is the possibility of the bladder being 'unsafe' and there is a risk of deterioration in kidney function.

– UDS should be performed according to ICS *Good Urodynamic Practice* 2016, with constant communication with the patient – to determine whether his/her everyday LUTS are reproduced and to correlate sensation with urodynamic findings – and using the event marker on the urodynamic machine.

– An established methodology should be used. Currently, this involves the use of water-filled catheters during pressure recording. The Working Group members have looked at the evidence for the clinical effectiveness of air-filled catheters, and do not recommend their use until there is an adequate evidence base of validation of the recordings obtained by this methodology.

– Perform those tests needed according to the individual patient and the clinical questions that have been asked. Tests may include urine flow study and measurement of PVR; filling cystometry; pressure-flow studies of voiding; urethral function studies; VUDS; and ambulatory UDS.

. *Urodynamic report:* the trace should be analysed and the main urodynamic pressure and flow findings documented. Any report should include the following:

– Name of referring clinician, and name and title of person performing the test
– Patient history, including allergies, last menstrual period, pregnancy status (if applicable)
– UDS urinalysis result and findings on physical examination
– Free flow data and any initial PVR
– Catheters used including size, and the filling rate and position of patient during filling and voiding
– Bladder and urethral sensation, and pressure data recorded during both filling and voiding, together with cystometric capacity
– Type of any leakage seen during filling
– Urine flow as part of the pressure-flow study of voiding, voided volume and PVR
– The urodynamic diagnoses during filling and voiding, whether normal or abnormal
– For every patient, it should be documented whether their everyday symptoms were reproduced, either fully or partly, or were not reproduced, and if the UD questions were answered.

• *Discussion of urodynamic findings and outline of possible future management with the patient.* UDS are unlike most other patients' tests in view of the essential interaction that occurs between the patient and the clinician during UDS. As a result, the patient will expect and appreciate a discussion with the clinician after the test.

- *Ongoing care* after UDS includes: advising the patient to drink 500 ml–1 l of fluid as soon as he or she gets home, and to maintain a high fluid intake for 24 hours, with the aim of minimising the chance of a UTI; a statement as to the next step in their management; patients appreciate a copy of both the urodynamic report and the letter to the referring doctor; and seek the patient's experience where possible after UDS.

12.6 Urodynamic Techniques

This section sets out the skills that are required to deliver safe and effective UDS that benefit the patient by providing information, not otherwise available, to guide their future effective management. These skills are both *technical* and *clinical* and are needed to deliver an individualised test whist assuring quality standards are met leading to the accurate, clinically relevant, interpretation of the test.

Quality of urodynamic recordings is of fundamental importance, because a poor quality study is of no use and, at worst, might be interpreted wrongly and the patient's treatment misdirected. Table 12.2 gives the key measures by which quality can be assessed.

12.7 Urine Flow Studies and the Measurement of Post-void Residual Urine

- *Introduction:* Urine flow studies (UFS) are the simplest studies of voiding function, and it is considered mandatory to include the measurement of PVR. Patients presenting to the outpatient clinic with bothersome LUTS are usually asked to provide a urine sample for dipstick testing as a first-line basic screening assessment. This can mean that it is difficult for the patient to have an adequately filled bladder for UFS at the same clinic appointment. For this reason, many urological departments run a dedicated flow clinic. The largest group of patients undergoing UFS is men with LUTS presumed secondary to benign prostatic obstruction (BPO); however, this study is also an important initial investigation in females with voiding symptoms.

UFS are screening studies, without high diagnostic specificity. Their limitations are due to urine flow being a product of the propulsive forces generated by the bladder and the resistance to flow from the bladder outlet. Hence, low flow may be due to bladder outlet obstruction (BOO), or to detrusor muscle underactivity, or to a combination of the two.

- *Indications are to screen for:* dysfunctional voiding in children; low flow prior to SUI surgery in women with voiding symptoms; voiding difficulties in women, including women with possible obstruction due to pelvic organ prolapse; and low flow in men with LUTS possibly due to BPO.
- *Technical skill requirements:*
  - To understand the principles by which uroflowmeters and ultrasound (US) scanners work.
  - To be able to clean and maintain uroflowmeters and ultrasound machines.
  - To be able to carry out calibration checks on the uroflowmeter.
  - To recognise uroflowmetry trace artefacts.
  - To understand the relevant measurements which must be made and documented to ensure complete information is acquired.

- *Clinical skill requirements:*
  . To know the indications for uroflowmetry and PVR measurement.
  . To be able to provide clear instructions to the patient regarding the performance of the test.
  . To understand how the uroflowmeter and ultrasound (US) machine function, and the principles of calibration.
  . To understand the cause of uroflowmetry trace artefacts, and to prevent them where possible.
  . To try to ensure that an adequate voided volume is passed during uroflowmetry.
  . To understand the importance of bladder diary data in interpreting the UFS.
  . To establish whether the UFS was typical for the patient.
  . To broadly categorise flow studies into normal, characteristic of urethral stricture, suggestive of bladder outlet obstruction or detrusor underactivity, or other abnormal pattern.
  . To be able to issue a report detailing relevant history, any relevant physical findings, the measurements from the UFS, and the interpretation of the investigation together with any shortcomings of the individual's test, such as low voided volumes when there is no significant PVR.

- *Special considerations in:*
  . *Children:* often attend flow clinics with incompletely filled bladders, and pre-scanning with the handheld bladder scanner is useful to document the bladder size before asking the child to void. If the bladder is under-filled, some degree of flexibility is then required to allow the child to drink and then undertake the study quickly if/when the child has a strong desire to void. ICCS guidelines are followed. Voided volumes should be greater than 50% of functional bladder capacity. As a general rule, the square of the maximum flow rate $(Q_{max})^2$ should be greater than the voided volume.
  . *Women:* in women with POP, consider reducing the prolapse to assess voiding.
  . *Men:* clear instructions should be given to men prior to uroflowmetry in order to avoid potential artefacts arising from excessive movement of the urinary stream across the collecting funnel.
  . *Neurological:* many neurological patients are unable to void voluntarily and therefore are unable to do UFS.

12.8 Standard UDS: Filling Cystometry and Pressure-Flow Studies of Voiding

- *Introduction:* Standard UDS are the most frequently indicated type of UDS performed, which assess both the filling and the voiding phases of the micturition cycle. The principal aims are to define detrusor and urethral function during both filling and voiding phases. The bladder is almost always filled through a urethral catheter, whilst the pressures in both the bladder and the rectum (or vagina) are measured. Standard UDS are used when simultaneous imaging of anatomy is unlikely to be relevant.

- *Common indications:*

  - In women prior to stress urinary incontinence (SUI) surgery, to confirm the diagnosis and to establish whether there are any factors that may mitigate against an optimal outcome.
  - In women with bothersome voiding symptoms, in order to establish, if possible, the cause.
  - In men with bothersome voiding symptoms, in order to establish the potential diagnosis of bladder outlet obstruction, particularly if LUTS persist despite non-surgical therapies, and when surgical treatment for BPO is being considered.
  - In both men and women with persistent storage LUTS despite non-surgical therapies, most commonly for OAB when surgical treatment is being considered, such as sacral nerve stimulation or injection of botulinum toxin.
  - Patients refractory to conservative and medical therapies but remain bothered by symptoms and who are willing to consider invasive therapy.
  - In general, VUDS are the preferred UD test in children and neurological patients.

- *Technical skill requirements:*

  - To understand the principles of how the uroflowmeter and urodynamic equipment function, and their vulnerabilities, for example, excess pressure on a pressure transducer.
  - To be able to clean and maintain the uroflowmeter and urodynamic equipment.
  - To be able to perform calibration checks on the uroflowmeter, the pressure transducers and the bladder filling pump.
  - To assess the quality of the urodynamic recording during the test and to improve the quality if necessary.
  - To recognise and know the cause of, and prevent where possible, artefacts on the UD trace.
  - To be able to read the tracing, and analyse and record the urodynamic measurements of flow pressure and bladder capacity, in the UD report.

- *Clinical skill requirements:*

  - To know the indications for standard UDS.
  - To be able to take a detailed history from the patient.
  - To confirm and document that the relevant physical examinations have taken place, and if competent, to carry out any examination that has not been previously recorded. If not competent to do this, to clearly state to the referring clinician, in the UD report, the examination that is still required.
  - To be able to provide clear instructions to the patient regarding the performance of the test.
  - To be able to pass the urodynamic catheters.
  - To understand how the uroflowmeter, urodynamic machine and the bladder filling pump function, and the principles of calibration for each.
  - To recognise and know the cause of urodynamic trace artefacts.
  - To know when and how to change the UD technique during the test, if indicated, for example, provocation testing or altering filling rate.

- To understand the importance of bladder diary data in interpreting the UDS.
- To establish whether the patient's experience of both the filling and voiding phases of their UDS was typical for them.
- To be able to interpret, and validate the urodynamic data from the UDS, and issue a report detailing relevant history, any relevant physical findings, and the measurements and diagnoses from the UDS, for example, using the Bladder Outlet Obstruction Index and the Bladder Contractility Index in men.
- Interpretation of the investigation in the light of the patient's symptoms, mentioning any shortcomings or quality issues of the individual's test.
- To manage any adverse reactions during the test and in the post-procedure period, e.g. vasovagal attack.
- Compliance with local infection control best practice.

- *Special considerations in:*
  Children: standard UDS are rarely performed in children. The majority undergo VUDS to allow maximum information to be obtained from the study.
  Women: if there is POP prolapse, reduction during urodynamics may be needed.
  Men: the voiding phase of the urodynamic study should be carried out with the man in his usual voiding position. For most men, this is in the standing position, but this may not always be the case and the preferred voiding position should be established before the study.
  Neurological: standard UDS may be used when anatomical abnormalities and upper tract deterioration are unlikely, for example in multiple sclerosis; however, many do require VUDS.

12.8.1 Urethral Function Studies

- *Introduction:* Urethral function studies are not widely used. The most frequently used tests are urethral pressure profilometry (UPP) and abdominal/valsalva leak point pressure (ALPP/VLPP) measurement in patients with stress incontinence. There is no clear evidence as to which test is most useful: the principal aim is to assess urethral function during storage.
- Detrusor leak point pressures (DLPP) are also occasionally measured.
- *Common indications include:* in *women*, prior to surgery for recurrent or persistent bothersome stress incontinence, for bothersome voiding symptoms and/or idiopathic urinary retention, to assess possible urethral sphincter overactivity, and suspected urethral relaxation incontinence; in *men* with post-prostatectomy stress incontinence to assess the degree of urethral sphincter weakness prior to possible incontinence surgery, and in younger men with voiding symptoms and low flow rates, who are unlikely to have prostatic obstruction, in order to identify the site of any obstruction and to assess possible urethral sphincter overactivity; in patients with poorly functioning artificial sphincters, to assess their function; and in *neurological* patients or those with poor bladder compliance whose upper urinary tracts may be at risk from high-pressure bladder filling ('unsafe bladders').
- *Technical skill requirements are:* to understand the principles of urethral function studies and equipment; be able to clean and maintain perfusion pump and withdrawal machine (profilometer); be able to check the calibration of the equipment; understand different

types of pressure measurement (solid state or water perfused) and their differences if more than one method is used; be able to undertake static and dynamic UPP, recognise and know the cause of, and prevent where possible, urethral function study artefacts; know the standard measurements to make and to document, e.g. functional profile length and maximum urethral closure pressure; and for fluid-filled catheter UPP, to understand the relationship between withdrawal rate, infusion rate, system compliance and the concomitant constraints.

- *Clinical skill requirements, to:* know the indications for urethral function studies; understand the principles of urethral function studies; know how the profilometer functions; have a knowledge of the characteristic normal traces obtained in men and women; and to recognise and know the cause of, and prevent where possible, urethral function study artefacts.

12.9 Video UDS (VUDS)

- *Introduction:* VUDS are performed when there is a likely patient benefit in having anatomical information during the UD test, as that information may make a difference to the decisions made for future management. The benefits of VUDS must be judged to be greater than the risks of irradiation to patients and staff, and the additional cost involved, and VUDS usually use X-ray fluoroscopic imaging, although ultrasound can be used.

- *Common indications:*

  - In children with congenital neurological conditions (e.g. spina bifida and sacral agenesis), congenital structural conditions (e.g. posterior urethral valves, bladder exstrophy), dysfunctional voiding and for failed OAB treatment prior to sacral nerve stimulation or BTXA.
  - In women, prior to possible repeat surgery for recurrent or persistent bothersome stress incontinence.
  - In women with urinary retention/incomplete emptying to provide information regarding the site of obstruction at bladder neck/mid-urethra/pelvic floor.
  - In younger men with voiding symptoms and low flow rates, who are less likely to have prostatic obstruction, in order to identify the site of any obstruction.
  - In men with post-prostatectomy stress incontinence prior to possible incontinence surgery.
  - In neurological patients where the upper tract is potentially at risk, due to an 'unsafe bladder', for example, in spinal cord injury and spina bifida.

- *Technical skill requirements:* VUDS require the same technical skill set needed for standard UDS and, in addition, staff should:

  - have had the radiological training in order to use the X-ray equipment, unless this is a responsibility of radiology staff;
  - have an understanding of the safety issues arising from video UDS using X-ray imaging;
  - know when and how to obtain the necessary images;
  - be able to reset the UD software to allow for the increased fluid density of contrast medium.

- *Clinical skill requirements:* VUDS require the same clinical skill set needed for standard UDS and, in addition, staff should:
  - have an understanding of the safety issues arising from VUDS using X-ray imaging;
  - ensure that all women under 55 years have an assessment of pregnancy/breast feeding status;
  - know when and how to obtain the necessary images;
  - have a detailed knowledge of the anatomy of the pelvic region;
  - know how to manage a reaction to contrast media.

- *Special considerations in children:*
  - The child must be prepared for the process of urethral (and rectal) catheterisation prior to the study. If the child has neurogenic LUTD, intermittent self-catheterisation (ISC) is likely to have been established already, and the urodynamics is generally well tolerated. If the child has idiopathic LUTD, then it is likely that they will need to undertake ISC in the future. In that situation, the urology nurse specialist will need to be closely involved with the family and home/hospital visits organised to try to establish ISC. If this proves impossible, then suprapubic urodynamic lines may need to be placed under general anaesthetic 24 hours prior to the study.
  - Most children prefer to sit for the study.
  - Distracting the child with cartoons/videos/games on iPad/tablet/phone may be useful.
  - Bladder capacity must be considered prior to starting the study (either functional from a bladder diary, or expected using standard formulae, e.g. capacity (ml) = (age in years × 30) + 30).
  - Fill rates should be low, generally 5–10 ml/min with an absolute maximum of 10% of bladder capacity per minute.
  - Video images should be taken regularly during the study.
  - The voiding phase may provide limited information in children, as children with neurogenic LUTD are generally unable to empty, and children with idiopathic LUTD may be unhappy to void with the urethral catheter in situ.

- *Special considerations in women:* the benefits of video must be clearly established in women of reproductive age. Local policy will likely require a pregnancy test, and if positive, will prevent X-ray from being used.

- *Special considerations in men:*
  - When anatomical details of the bladder neck and urethra are required, it may be necessary to position the male patient in the 30 degrees oblique position in order to avoid any potential artefact from the bony pelvis.
  - During provocation for suspected stress urinary incontinence in males, it is often necessary to carry out a second fill, following which the urodynamic catheters should be removed and the provocation repeated: the increase in outlet resistance, due to the presence of urodynamic catheters, can sometimes prevent the demonstration of mild urodynamic stress incontinence.

- *Special considerations in neurological patients:*
  - Health-care professionals should only undertake urodynamics on neurological patients if they understand the patient's condition, including hand function, and

mobility and cognition, and the potential effects these will have on the management of the patient's bladder and bowel function. They also need to understand the potential for progression and change to make the urodynamics meaningful. Neurological patients need an individualised study according to the urodynamic questions that need to be answered.

. Spinal injury patients with a level of T6 or above are at risk of autonomic dysreflexia and should only undergo urodynamics in a unit that is familiar with recognising and managing this condition.

. Safety issues that are most important in spinal cord injured patients: higher risk of *latex allergy* – the UDU should have a latex-free policy; attention needs to be paid to skin areas, particularly if the patient has a lack of sensation or skin breakage; assess the risk of *autonomic dysreflexia* – staff should know when to use prophylaxis and how to treat if it occurs.

. Practical issues include the following: *mobility* is often reduced and therefore the patient may need hoisting onto the UD table and *positioning* on the table may be difficult; recording flow in the *voiding phase* may not be possible, although, in men, a *drainpipe* may need to be used to measure leakage and collect voided urine; although most VUDS are done *supine,* some patients can stand.

. Urodynamic technique adaptations include the following: the bladder should be *emptied* if that patient would normally do so; those with a *suprapubic catheter* (SPC) should be filled, and pressure recorded, through the SPC; bladder filling should be done slowly, usually commencing at a rate of 20 ml/min; the *rectum should be emptied* if found to be loaded, as this can affect the recording of rectal (abdominal) pressure and detrusor function during voiding; and *DLPP* may need to be measured, and the effect that VUR may have on DLPP appreciated.

- If incontinence surgery is being considered, the bladder needs to be filled to the appropriate volume for that patient, and it may be necessary to obstruct the urethra to achieve this: in men, this can be performed by a penile clamp, and in women urethral compression may be needed.

12.10 Ambulatory UDS (AUDS)

- *Introduction:*

  . The aim of AUDS is to reproduce the patient's symptoms by allowing the patient to do those activities that cause the symptoms. During AUDS, the patient can move freely and leave the UDU returning to void.

  . Instead of artificial bladder filling, the bladder is filled naturally (physiologically) by the patient's own urine. Therefore, the average bladder filling rate is 60–120 ml/hour (1–2 ml/min). As with other UD techniques, both bladder and rectal or vaginal pressures are recorded throughout filling and voiding phases.

  . AUDS are performed in regional centres in a highly selected group of patients and require considerable additional time, resources and equipment which is specifically designed for this purpose.

- *Common indications:* Those patients with bothersome LUTS who have failed non-surgical treatments, but whose standard or video UDS have failed to reproduce the patient's symptoms, and therefore further treatment is being delayed whilst a clear cause for the LUTS is established.

- *Technical skill requirements:* Ambulatory UDS requires the same technical skill set needed for standard UDS and, in addition, staff should understand how the AUDS equipment functions, including use of solid-state, air-filled or water-filled catheters, and any sterilisation issues; be able to clean and maintain the AUDS equipment; be able to check calibration of the transducers and the AUDS machine; and recognise and know the cause of, and prevent where possible, AUDS artefacts.
- *Clinical skill requirements:* Ambulatory UDS requires the same clinical skill set needed for standard UDS (see Section 12.8), and, in addition, staff should:
    - Know the indications for ambulatory UDS.
    - Be able to adapt the test and the clinical environment to ensure the patient's symptoms/exacerbating conditions are recreated.
    - Be able to download and to analyse the AUDS recording.
    - Be able to use the urodynamic data from the AUDS, and issue a report detailing relevant history, any relevant physical findings, the measurements from the UDS, and the interpretation of the investigation together with any shortcomings of the individual's test.

- *Special considerations:* in children, although ambulatory UDS and natural bladder filling offer potential benefit in children, the equipment and expertise are only available in a very limited number of tertiary centres, and as a result, the technique has not been widely adopted.

12.11 General Recommendations

- UDS have become widely accepted as an essential investigation into LUTD over the last 40 years. However, there is no regulation with respect to the training of staff or assessment of quality in the performance of UDS. Hence, patients are at risk from sub-standard UD assessment, but are not aware of this regrettable omission. The UKCS considers that all UD staff should undergo formal training, and fulfill set CPD requirements in order to maintain their skills.
- All UDUs should have a designated suitably qualified director responsible for UD quality assurance, including UD audit, staff appointment and training, and the MDT process.
- High-quality UDS demand that the UD HCPs possess two essential skill sets, technical and clinical, and these are defined for the first time.
- The patient's UD pathway is defined, and integral to this is an appropriate UD referral and the systematic provision of full information to all patients.
- The requirements for the range of UD tests are defined, and the skill sets required to deliver a high-quality UDS are listed.
- This report provides the details required to ensure that the Commissioners know the necessary specification of the UD services that they are purchasing, and that the providers know the criteria they must meet when offering to provide a urodynamic service.

References

1. Working Group of the United Kingdom Continence Society; Abrams P, Eustice S, Gammie A, et al. United Kingdom Continence Society: Minimum standards for urodynamic studies, 2018. *Neurourol Urodyn.* 2019;38(2):838–56.

2. Abrams P, Cardozo L, Fall M, et al. The standardisation of terminology of lower urinary tract function: report from the Standardisation Sub-committee of the International Continence Society. *Neurourol Urodyn.* 2002;21(2):167–78.

3. Hogan S, Gammie A, Abrams P. Urodynamic features and artefacts. *Neurourol Urodyn.* 2012;31(7):1104–17.

4. Gammie A, Clarkson B, Constantinou C, et al. International Continence Society Urodynamic Equipment Working Group. International Continence Society guidelines on urodynamic equipment performance. *Neurourol Urodyn.* 2014;33:370–9.

5. Rosier P, Schaefer W, Lose G, et al. International Continence Society Good Urodynamic Practices and Terms 2016: urodynamics, uroflowmetry, cystometry, and pressure-flow study. *Neurourol Urodyn.* 2017;33(4):370.

6. Chapple CR, Hillary CJ, Patel A, MacDiarmid SA. *Urodynamics Made Easy.* E-Book. London: Churchill Livingstone; 2018.

7. Abrams P. *Urodynamics.* London: Springer; 2006.

8. Bauer SB, Nijman RJ, Drzewiecki BA, Sillen U, Hoebeke P; International Children's Continence Society Standardization Subcommittee. International Children's Continence Society standardization report on urodynamic studies of the lower urinary tract in children. *Neurourol Urodyn.* 2015;34:640–7.

9. Austin PF, Bauer SB, Bower W, et al. The standardisation of terminology of lower urinary tract function in children and adolescents: update report from the Standardisation Committee of the International Children's Continence Society. *Neurourol Urodyn.* 2016;35:471–81.

10. Mosiello G, Del Popolo G, Wen JG, De Gennaro M. *Clinical Urodynamics in Childhood and Adolescence.* Urodynamics, Neurourology and Pelvic Floor Dysfunctions. Cham: Springer; 2018.

Index

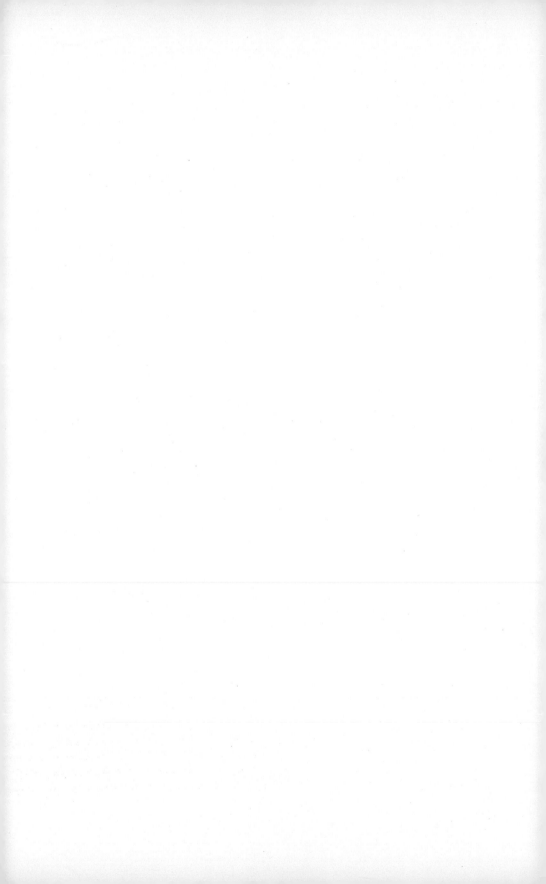